VEGETARIAN DIET COOKBOOK 2024

A Simple Guide to Creating Delicious and Nutritious Meals for Healthy Living

By

Hector Wiggins

Table of Contents

INTRODUCTION

Once upon a time, in kitchens around the world, a quiet revolution was taking place. It wasn't marked by protests or grand declarations, but rather by the gentle sizzle of vegetables in a pan and the satisfying aroma of spices dancing in the air. This revolution was the rise of the vegetarian diet – a movement fueled not only by compassion for animals but also by a growing awareness of the impact our food choices have on the planet and our own well-being.

In this cookbook, we embark on a culinary journey that celebrates the beauty and bounty of plant-based eating. Welcome to the Vegetarian Diet Cookbook of 2024, where each recipe is a love letter to nature's vibrant palette and a testament to the endless possibilities of meat-free cuisine.

Picture yourself standing in a bustling farmer's market, surrounded by crates overflowing with freshly picked produce – ruby-red tomatoes, emerald-green kale, golden ears of corn. These are the ingredients that form the foundation of our recipes, each one carefully selected for its flavor, nutrition, and sustainability.

But this cookbook is more than just a collection of recipes; it's a celebration of creativity and exploration in the kitchen. Whether you're a seasoned chef or a novice cook, there's something here for everyone – from quick and easy weeknight meals to elaborate feasts fit for a special occasion.

As we turn the pages of this book, we'll discover the art of transforming humble ingredients into culinary masterpieces. We'll learn the secrets of building layers of flavor, balancing textures and colors, and creating dishes that not only nourish the body but also delight the senses.

But our journey doesn't stop at the kitchen door. Throughout these pages, we'll also explore the broader implications of our food choices – from the environmental impact of industrial farming to the ethical considerations of animal agriculture. We'll discuss the health benefits of a plant-based diet, backed by scientific research and real-life testimonials.

So, whether you're here to expand your culinary horizons, improve your health, or do your part to protect the planet, know that you're not alone. Together, we can create a world where every meal is a celebration of life, love, and the power of plants. So let's roll up our sleeves, sharpen our knives, and embark on this delicious adventure together. The green plate awaits – let's dig in!

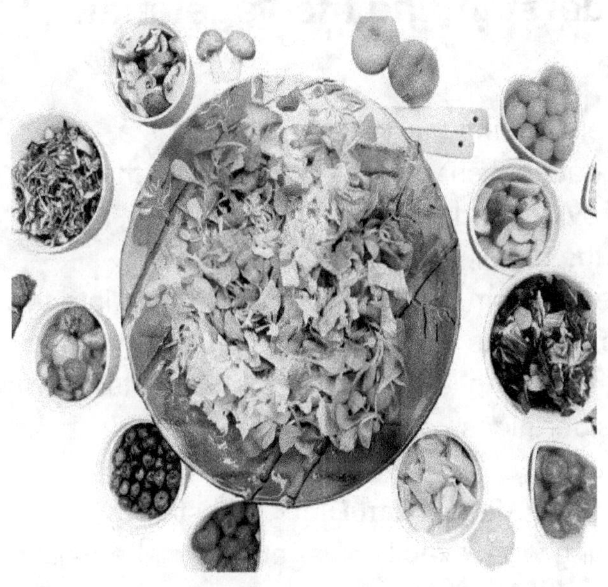

Understanding the Vegetarian Diet

Understanding the Vegetarian Diet" is a foundational chapter in our cookbook that aims to provide readers with comprehensive insights into the principles and nuances of vegetarianism. In this section, we delve into the core concepts of what constitutes a vegetarian diet, exploring its various forms, benefits, and considerations.

What is a Vegetarian Diet?: We start by defining what exactly a vegetarian diet entails. This includes abstaining from consuming meat, poultry, and seafood, while embracing a diverse array of plant-based foods such as fruits, vegetables, grains, legumes, nuts, and seeds.

Benefits of a Vegetarian Lifestyle: Next, we highlight the numerous benefits associated with adopting a vegetarian lifestyle. These benefits extend beyond personal health to encompass environmental sustainability, animal welfare, and even social justice. By reducing our reliance on animal products, we can decrease our carbon footprint, alleviate animal suffering, and promote a more equitable food system.

Types of Vegetarian Diets: We then explore the different variations of the vegetarian diet, acknowledging that there is no one-size-fits-all approach. From lacto-ovo vegetarians who include dairy and eggs in their diet to vegans who eschew all animal-derived products, each dietary preference comes with its own set of considerations and nutritional considerations.

Through "Understanding the Vegetarian Diet," readers gain a deeper appreciation for the principles underlying vegetarianism, empowering them to make informed choices about their dietary habits. Whether they're seasoned vegetarians looking to expand their culinary repertoire or curious omnivores exploring plant-based options, this chapter serves as a valuable resource for understanding and embracing the vegetarian lifestyle.

What is a Vegetarian Diet

A vegetarian diet is a dietary pattern that primarily consists of plant-based foods and excludes meat, poultry, and seafood. Vegetarians typically consume a variety of fruits, vegetables, grains, legumes, nuts, seeds, and plant-based protein sources. There are different variations of the vegetarian diet, including:

Lacto-ovo Vegetarian: This diet includes dairy products () and eggs (ovo) but excludes meat, poultry, and seafood.

Lacto-Vegetarian: Similar to lacto-ovo vegetarians, but excludes eggs while including dairy products.

Ovo-Vegetarian: Includes eggs but excludes dairy products.

Vegan: A strict plant-based diet that excludes all animal-derived products, including dairy, eggs, honey, and sometimes even certain additives and ingredients derived from animals.

Vegetarians choose this dietary lifestyle for various reasons, including health benefits, environmental sustainability, ethical concerns related to animal welfare, and personal preferences. A well-planned vegetarian diet can provide ample nutrients such as fiber, vitamins, minerals, and antioxidants while reducing the consumption of saturated fats and cholesterol found in animal products.

Benefits of a Vegetarian Lifestyle

The benefits of adopting a vegetarian lifestyle are multifaceted and extend beyond individual health to encompass environmental sustainability, animal welfare, and even social justice. Here are some key benefits:

Improved Health: Numerous studies have shown that vegetarian diets are associated with lower risks of chronic diseases such as heart disease, hypertension, type 2 diabetes, and certain cancers. Vegetarian diets are typically higher in fiber, vitamins, minerals, and antioxidants, while lower in saturated fats and cholesterol found in animal products. This can contribute to better overall health and longevity.

Environmental Sustainability: Deforestation, water pollution, greenhouse gas emissions, and habitat degradation are all directly caused by animal husbandry. We can mitigate our influence on the environment by consuming fewer or no animal products. Plant-based diets are more environmentally friendly and sustainable since they use less land, water, and grain.

Animal care: Living a vegetarian lifestyle is consistent with moral principles pertaining to the rights and care of animals. Animals raised in factories are frequently subjected to cruel treatment, overcrowding, and confinement. People can lessen the need for animals raised in factories and contribute to the relief of animal suffering by making plant-based dietary choices.

Social Justice: Vegetarianism can intersect with social justice issues, such as food accessibility and global hunger. Plant-based diets require fewer resources to produce, making them a more efficient way to feed a growing global population. By reducing our reliance on animal agriculture, we can allocate resources more equitably and address food insecurity more effectively.

Weight Management: Vegetarian diets are often associated with lower body weight and body mass index (BMI), as they tend to be lower in calories and saturated fats compared to omnivorous diets. Plant-based foods are also higher in fiber, which can promote feelings of fullness and aid in weight management.

Improved Digestion: The high fiber content of vegetarian diets can promote healthy digestion and bowel movements, reducing the risk of constipation and promoting gut health.

Overall, adopting a vegetarian lifestyle offers a myriad of benefits for both individuals and the planet, promoting health, sustainability, and compassion.

Types of Vegetarian Diets

The word "vegetarian" refers to a range of dietary regimens that forgo different kinds of animal products. The primary kinds of vegetarian diets are as follows:

The most popular kind of vegetarian diet is lacto-ovo vegetarianism. Vegetarians who follow the lacto-ovo diet do not consume any meat, poultry, or seafood; instead, they consume dairy and eggs. This diet is quite simple to stick to and offers a large variety of food selections.

Lacto-Vegetarian: Lacto-vegetarians exclude meat, poultry, seafood, and eggs from their diet but include dairy products such as milk, cheese, yogurt, and butter. They derive their protein and calcium primarily from dairy sources.

Ovo-Vegetarian: Ovo-vegetarians exclude meat, poultry, seafood, and dairy products from their diet but include eggs. They may consume foods like tofu, tempeh, legumes, grains, fruits, vegetables, and plant-based milk alternatives.

Vegan: Vegans adhere to a strict plant-based diet that excludes all animal-derived products, including meat, poultry, seafood, dairy, eggs, honey, and other animal by-products. They rely solely on plant-based foods for their nutrition and may also avoid products tested on animals and clothing made from animal materials.

Flexitarian or Semi-Vegetarian: Flexitarians primarily follow a vegetarian diet but occasionally include small amounts of meat, poultry, or seafood in their meals. They emphasize plant-based foods but are flexible in their dietary choices.

These different types of vegetarian diets offer individuals flexibility in choosing a dietary pattern that aligns with their health goals, ethical beliefs, cultural practices, and personal preferences. Regardless of the specific type, all vegetarian diets prioritize plant-based foods and exclude or limit the consumption of animal products.

CHAPTER ONE

Breakfast Recipes

Breakfast Recipes" is a section in our vegetarian diet cookbook dedicated to providing a diverse array of nutritious and delicious morning meal options that align with a plant-based lifestyle. Here's a comprehensive overview of what readers can expect from this section:

Variety of Options: The Breakfast Recipes section offers a wide variety of options to suit different tastes and preferences. From savory to sweet, light to hearty, and quick to more elaborate, there's something for everyone to enjoy.

Nutrient-Rich Ingredients: Each recipe is carefully crafted to incorporate nutrient-rich ingredients that provide essential vitamins, minerals, and antioxidants to kickstart the day. Ingredients such as whole grains, fruits, vegetables, nuts, seeds, and plant-based protein sources are prominently featured.

Balanced Nutrition: The recipes in this section are designed to provide balanced nutrition, including a good balance of carbohydrates, protein, and healthy fats. This helps to keep readers feeling satisfied and energized throughout the morning.

Ease of Preparation: Many of the breakfast recipes are designed to be quick and easy to prepare, making them perfect for busy weekday mornings. Simple techniques and minimal ingredients are emphasized to streamline the cooking process without compromising on flavor or nutrition.

Creative and Flavorful Dishes: While some recipes may be classic breakfast staples with a vegetarian twist, others showcase innovative flavor combinations and culinary techniques. Readers can expect to discover new and exciting flavor profiles that challenge traditional notions of breakfast.

Customizable Options: Most recipes offer suggestions for customization to accommodate individual dietary preferences and ingredient availability. Whether readers are looking to add extra protein, incorporate seasonal produce, or adjust the flavor profile to suit their taste buds, there's room for creativity and personalization.

Inspiration for Special Occasions: While many of the recipes are suitable for everyday breakfasts, there are also options that can elevate special occasions or leisurely weekend brunches. These recipes may be more elaborate or indulgent, offering readers an opportunity to celebrate and savor the morning moments.

Overall, the Breakfast Recipes section of our vegetarian diet cookbook aims to inspire readers to start their day on a nutritious and satisfying note, showcasing the versatility and deliciousness of plant-based breakfast options. Whether readers are seasoned vegetarians or new to the lifestyle, this section provides a wealth of inspiration and practical guidance for creating wholesome and flavorful morning meals.

Classic Veggie Omelette

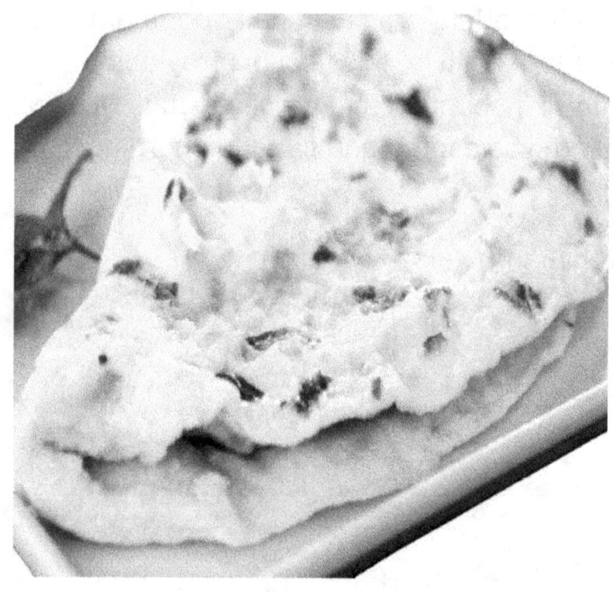

The Classic Veggie Omelette is a staple breakfast dish in vegetarian cuisine, offering a nutritious and satisfying way to start the day. Here's a comprehensive explanation of what this dish entails:

Ingredients: The Classic Veggie Omelette typically consists of eggs, a variety of vegetables, cheese (optional), herbs, and seasonings. Common vegetables used in this dish include bell peppers, onions, mushrooms, tomatoes, spinach, and zucchini, but the choice of vegetables can vary based on personal preference and seasonal availability.

Preparation: To prepare the Classic Veggie Omelette, start by whisking eggs together in a bowl until they are well beaten. Meanwhile, sauté the chopped vegetables in a skillet with a little oil or butter until they are tender and slightly caramelized.

Once the vegetables are cooked, pour the beaten eggs over the vegetables in the skillet and allow them to cook undisturbed until the edges start to set.

Folding Technique: Once the edges of the omelet are set, use a spatula to gently lift the edges of the omelet and allow any uncooked egg to flow underneath. When the eggs are mostly set but still slightly runny on top, sprinkle cheese (if using) over one half of the omelet and fold the other half over the filling. Let the omelet cook for another minute or so until the cheese is melted and the eggs are fully cooked through.

Presentation: Carefully slide the cooked omelet onto a plate and garnish with fresh herbs, such as parsley or chives, for added flavor and visual appeal. The omelet can be served hot and fluffy, with the cheese oozing out of the center and the vegetables peeking through.

Customization: The beauty of the Classic Veggie Omelette lies in its versatility and adaptability. Feel free to customize the recipe based on personal taste preferences and ingredient availability. You can add additional ingredients such as diced ham, tofu, or avocado for added protein and texture, or experiment with different herbs and spices to elevate the flavor profile.

Nutritional Benefits: This vegetarian omelet is not only delicious but also nutritious, providing a good balance of protein, vitamins, minerals, and fiber from the eggs and vegetables. It's a satisfying and wholesome breakfast option that can keep you fueled and energized throughout the morning.

Overall, the Classic Veggie Omelette is a timeless breakfast favorite that celebrates the flavors and versatility of vegetarian cooking. Whether enjoyed as a quick weekday breakfast or a leisurely weekend brunch, this dish is sure to please vegetarians and non-vegetarians alike with its simplicity, flavor, and nourishment.

Avocado Toast with Tomato and Basil

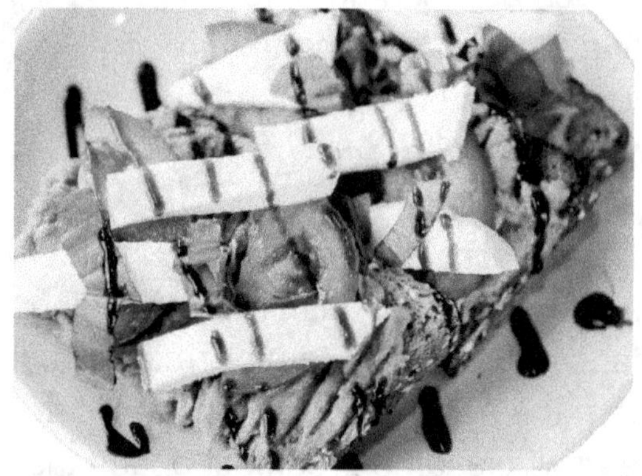

Avocado Toast with Tomato and Basil is a popular and nutritious breakfast or snack option that is perfect for vegetarians. Here's a comprehensive explanation of what this dish entails:

Ingredients: Avocado Toast with Tomato and Basil typically consists of a few simple ingredients:

Bread: Choose your favorite type of bread, such as whole wheat, sourdough, or multigrain.

Avocado: Ripe avocados are mashed and spread onto the toast as a creamy base.

Tomato: Fresh, ripe tomatoes are sliced and layered on top of the mashed avocado.

Basil: Fresh basil leaves add a burst of flavor and aroma to the dish.

Optional toppings: Additional toppings such as red onion slices, microgreens, lemon juice, balsamic glaze, or crushed red pepper flakes can be added for extra flavor and texture.

Preparation: To make Avocado Toast with Tomato and Basil, start by toasting the bread until golden brown and crisp. While the bread is toasting, mash the avocado in a bowl with a fork until smooth and creamy. Once the bread is toasted, spread the mashed avocado evenly onto the toast slices.

Assembly: Layer the sliced tomatoes on top of the mashed avocado, arranging them in a single layer for even distribution. Next, tear or chiffonade the fresh basil leaves and sprinkle them generously over the tomatoes. For added flavor, drizzle a little olive oil and season with salt and pepper to taste.

Presentation: Arrange the prepared avocado toast slices on a serving platter or individual plates. Garnish with additional basil leaves or other optional toppings for a visually appealing presentation.

Customization: Avocado Toast with Tomato and Basil is highly customizable, allowing you to tailor the dish to your taste preferences and dietary needs. You can experiment with different types of bread, add extra toppings such as sliced cucumbers or radishes, or incorporate a squeeze of lemon juice or a sprinkle of nutritional yeast for added flavor.

Nutritional Benefits: This dish is not only delicious but also nutritious, providing a good balance of healthy fats, fiber, vitamins, and minerals. Avocados are rich in monounsaturated fats, which are heart-healthy, while tomatoes are packed with vitamins C and K, as well as antioxidants. Basil adds a refreshing herbal note and is a good source of vitamin K and manganese.

Overall, Avocado Toast with Tomato and Basil is a simple yet satisfying dish that celebrates the flavors of fresh, wholesome ingredients. Whether enjoyed for breakfast, brunch, or as a quick and healthy snack, this vegetarian dish is sure to become a favorite in your culinary repertoire.

Blueberry Spinach Smoothie Bowl

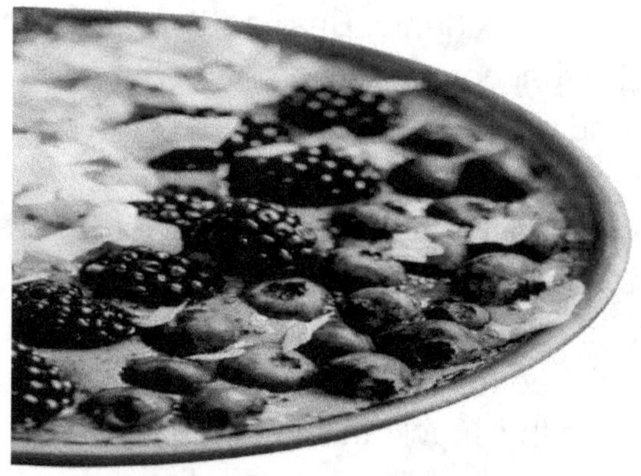

Blueberry Spinach Smoothie Bowl is a nutritious and delicious breakfast or snack option that is perfect for vegetarians. Here's a comprehensive explanation of what this dish entails:

Ingredients: The Blueberry Spinach Smoothie Bowl typically consists of the following ingredients:

Frozen blueberries: Blueberries are rich in antioxidants, vitamins, and minerals, making them a nutritious addition to the smoothie bowl. Fresh spinach: Spinach adds a vibrant green color and a boost of nutrients, including vitamins A, C, and K, as well as iron and folate.
Banana: Ripe banana adds natural sweetness and creaminess to the smoothie bowl while providing potassium, fiber, and other essential nutrients.
Greek yogurt or plant-based yogurt: Yogurt adds creaminess and protein to the smoothie bowl, contributing to its satisfying texture and nutritional profile.

Liquid: Liquid such as almond milk, coconut water, or plain water is added to achieve the desired consistency of the smoothie bowl.

Toppings: Toppings such as fresh berries, sliced banana, granola, chia seeds, shredded coconut, or nuts can be added for extra flavor, texture, and nutritional benefits.

Preparation: To make the Blueberry Spinach Smoothie Bowl, start by blending the frozen blueberries, fresh spinach, ripe banana, yogurt, and liquid of choice in a high-speed blender until smooth and creamy. Adjust the amount of liquid as needed to achieve the desired consistency – thicker for a spoonable smoothie bowl or thinner for a drinkable smoothie.

Assembly: Pour the blended smoothie into a bowl and use a spoon to smooth the surface. Arrange the desired toppings on top of the smoothie bowl in an attractive and visually appealing manner.

Feel free to get creative with the toppings, adding a variety of colors, textures, and flavors to enhance the overall experience.

Presentation: Serve the Blueberry Spinach Smoothie Bowl immediately, garnished with additional fresh berries, herbs, or a drizzle of honey if desired. The vibrant colors and enticing presentation make this smoothie bowl a feast for the eyes as well as the taste buds.

Nutritional Benefits: This smoothie bowl is not only delicious but also packed with essential nutrients, including vitamins, minerals, fiber, and antioxidants. Blueberries and spinach are both nutrient-dense superfoods that offer numerous health benefits, while banana adds natural sweetness and creaminess without the need for added sugars. Greek yogurt or plant-based yogurt provides protein and probiotics, promoting gut health and satiety.

Overall, the Blueberry Spinach Smoothie Bowl is a nutritious and satisfying vegetarian option that offers a delicious way to incorporate more fruits and vegetables into your diet. Whether enjoyed for breakfast, as a post-workout snack, or as a refreshing treat on a hot day, this smoothie bowl is sure to leave you feeling nourished and energized.

CHAPTER TWO

Appetizers and Snacks

"Appetizers and Snacks" in a vegetarian diet cookbook offers a delightful array of finger foods and small bites that are perfect for entertaining guests, satisfying hunger between meals, or simply indulging in a flavorful snack. Here's a comprehensive explanation of what this section entails:

Variety of Options: The Appetizers and Snacks section offers a wide variety of options to suit different tastes, occasions, and dietary preferences. From light and refreshing appetizers to savory and satisfying snacks, there's something for every palate and craving.

Plant-Based Ingredients: All the recipes in this section are entirely plant-based, meaning they exclude meat, poultry, seafood, and any other animal-derived ingredients. Instead, they rely on a diverse range of plant-based ingredients such as fruits, vegetables, grains, legumes, nuts, seeds, herbs, and spices.

Nutrient-Rich and Flavorful: Despite being vegetarian, the appetizers and snacks in this section are packed with flavor, texture, and nutrition. They showcase the versatility and deliciousness of plant-based ingredients, highlighting their ability to create satisfying and appetizing dishes without the need for meat or animal products.

Easy Preparation: Many of the recipes in this section are designed to be quick and easy to prepare, making them ideal for busy lifestyles or last-minute entertaining.

Simple techniques and minimal ingredients are emphasized to streamline the cooking process and ensure that even novice cooks can achieve impressive results.

Great for Sharing: Appetizers and snacks are inherently social foods, meant to be shared and enjoyed with friends, family, or guests. Whether you're hosting a dinner party, potluck, or casual gathering, these vegetarian options provide a delicious and inclusive way to cater to diverse dietary needs and preferences.

Versatility and Adaptability: The recipes in this section are highly versatile and adaptable, allowing for customization based on personal taste preferences, ingredient availability, and dietary restrictions. Readers are encouraged to experiment with different flavor combinations, substitutions, and variations to suit their individual preferences and creativity.

Health Benefits: Vegetarian appetizers and snacks offer numerous health benefits, including being rich in fiber, vitamins, minerals, and antioxidants while typically being lower in saturated fats and cholesterol compared to meat-based alternatives. They provide a satisfying and nourishing way to curb hunger and boost energy levels throughout the day.

Hummus Trio Platter

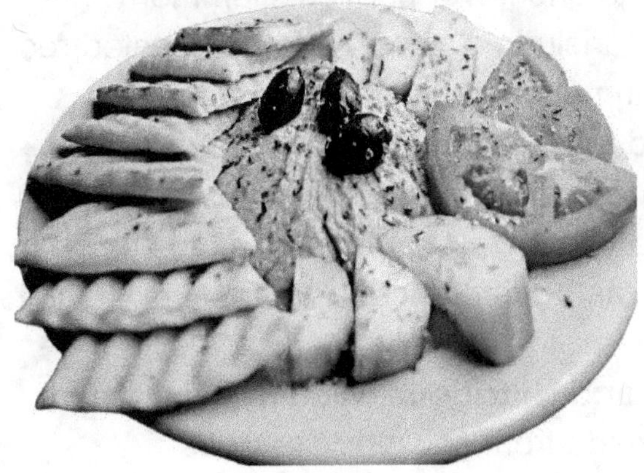

The Hummus Trio Platter is a delightful appetizer option in a vegetarian diet cookbook, offering a colorful array of creamy, flavorful hummus varieties served alongside an assortment of accompaniments. Here's a comprehensive explanation of what this dish entails:

Variety of Hummus Flavors: The Hummus Trio Platter typically features three different flavors of hummus, each showcasing unique ingredients and flavor profiles. Common variations include classic hummus, roasted red pepper hummus, garlic and herb hummus, sun-dried tomato hummus, spicy hummus, or avocado hummus. These variations add depth and variety to the platter, appealing to a wide range of taste preferences.

Creamy and Nutritious: Hummus is a creamy spread made from cooked chickpeas (garbanzo beans), tahini (ground sesame seeds), olive oil, lemon juice, garlic, and various seasonings. It is naturally vegan and rich in protein, fiber, healthy fats, vitamins, and minerals. Hummus is not only delicious but also nutritious, making it a perfect addition to a vegetarian diet.

Accompaniments: Alongside the hummus varieties, the platter typically includes an assortment of accompaniments for dipping and scooping. Common accompaniments may include:

Fresh vegetables: Crisp and colorful vegetables such as carrot sticks, cucumber slices, bell pepper strips, cherry tomatoes, and celery sticks add crunch and freshness to the platter.

Pita bread or crackers: Soft and fluffy pita bread, toasted pita wedges, or a selection of crackers provide a hearty base for scooping up the creamy hummus.

Olives: Briny and savory olives, such as Kalamata or green olives, add a burst of flavor and texture to the platter.

Pickled vegetables: Tangy and crunchy pickled vegetables, such as pickles, pickled onions, or pickled peppers, complement the creamy hummus with their acidity and bite.
Fresh herbs: Sprigs of fresh herbs, such as parsley, cilantro, or dill, add a pop of color and herbal freshness to the platter.
Presentation: The Hummus Trio Platter is typically arranged on a large serving platter or board, with each hummus flavor nestled in its own bowl or compartment. The accompaniments are arranged around the hummus, creating an attractive and inviting presentation that is perfect for sharing with friends, family, or guests.

Versatility and Customization: The beauty of the Hummus Trio Platter lies in its versatility and customization. Readers can mix and match their favorite hummus flavors and accompaniments to create a platter that suits their taste preferences and dietary needs.

The platter can be tailored to accommodate gluten-free, dairy-free, or other dietary restrictions with ease.

Overall, the Hummus Trio Platter is a delicious and nutritious appetizer option that celebrates the flavors and versatility of hummus in vegetarian cuisine. Whether enjoyed as a starter for a dinner party, a snack for game day, or a light meal on its own, this platter is sure to impress with its vibrant colors, bold flavors, and wholesome ingredients.

Stuffed Mini Bell Peppers

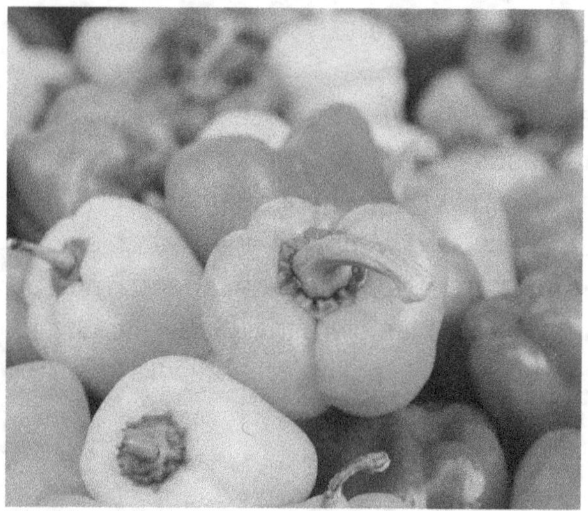

Stuffed Mini Bell Peppers are a delightful and versatile appetizer option in a vegetarian diet, offering a colorful and flavorful way to enjoy fresh bell peppers. Here's a comprehensive explanation of what this dish entails:

Ingredients: Stuffed Mini Bell Peppers typically consist of the following ingredients:

Mini bell peppers: Small bell peppers are halved and hollowed out to create cups for the filling. Their vibrant colors – red, yellow, orange, and green – add visual appeal to the dish.

Filling ingredients: The filling often includes a combination of cooked grains (such as quinoa, rice, or couscous), protein-rich ingredients (such as beans, lentils, tofu, or tempeh), vegetables (such as onions, garlic, corn, tomatoes, spinach, or mushrooms), herbs (such as parsley, basil, or cilantro), and seasonings (such as salt, pepper, cumin, paprika, or chili powder).

Optional toppings: Toppings such as shredded cheese (vegan or dairy-based), breadcrumbs, or fresh herbs can be added for extra flavor, texture, and visual appeal.

Preparation: To make Stuffed Mini Bell Peppers, start by halving the mini bell peppers lengthwise and removing the seeds and membranes to create hollow cups. Next, prepare the filling by cooking the grains, protein, and vegetables separately, then combining them with herbs and seasonings in a bowl. Spoon the filling mixture into the hollowed-out bell pepper halves until they are generously filled.

Baking or Grilling: The stuffed bell peppers can be baked in the oven or grilled on the barbecue until the peppers are tender and the filling is heated through and slightly golden brown on top. Baking typically takes about 15-20 minutes at 375°F (190°C), while grilling may take slightly less time depending on the temperature of the grill.

Presentation: Once cooked, arrange the Stuffed Mini Bell Peppers on a serving platter or baking dish. Garnish with optional toppings such as shredded cheese, breadcrumbs, or fresh herbs for added flavor and visual appeal.

Versatility and Customization: The beauty of Stuffed Mini Bell Peppers lies in their versatility and adaptability. Readers can customize the filling based on personal taste preferences, ingredient availability, and dietary restrictions. The filling can be adjusted to accommodate vegan, gluten-free, dairy-free, or other dietary preferences with ease.

Nutritional Benefits: Stuffed Mini Bell Peppers are not only delicious but also nutritious, providing a good balance of carbohydrates, protein, fiber, vitamins, and minerals.

Bell peppers are rich in vitamin C, vitamin A, and antioxidants, while the filling ingredients contribute additional nutrients and flavor to the dish. This makes Stuffed Mini Bell Peppers a satisfying and wholesome appetizer option that is perfect for vegetarians and non-vegetarians alike.

Overall, Stuffed Mini Bell Peppers are a delightful and versatile appetizer option in a vegetarian diet cookbook, offering a colorful and flavorful way to enjoy fresh bell peppers. Whether served as an appetizer for a dinner party, a side dish for a barbecue, or a light meal on their own, these stuffed peppers are sure to impress with their vibrant colors, bold flavors, and wholesome ingredients.

Vegan Cheese and Crackers Board

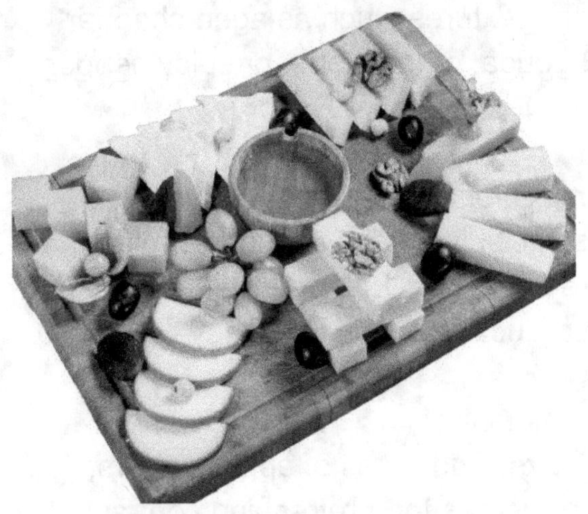

A Vegan Cheese and Crackers Board for a vegetarian diet typically consists of a variety of dairy-free cheeses, crackers, and complementary accompaniments. Here's a comprehensive breakdown:

Dairy-Free Cheeses: Select a variety of vegan cheeses made from nuts (like cashews or almonds), soy, coconut, or other plant-based ingredients. These cheeses come in different flavors and textures, such as aged cheddar, smoked gouda, creamy brie, or spicy pepper jack.

Crackers: Offer an assortment of vegan crackers, including plain, seeded, whole grain, or flavored varieties. Ensure they are free from animal products like dairy or honey.

Accompaniments:
Fresh Fruits: Add slices of apples, pears, grapes, or berries for a refreshing contrast to the savory cheeses and crackers.
Dried Fruits: Include dried apricots, figs, or cranberries for a sweet and chewy element.
Nuts and Seeds: Offer a mix of raw or roasted nuts like almonds, walnuts, or pistachios, as well as seeds like pumpkin or sunflower seeds for added crunch and protein.

Olives: Include a variety of olives for a salty and briny component.

Pickles: Add some pickled vegetables like cucumbers, carrots, or cauliflower for tanginess.

Jams or Chutneys: Offer small bowls of vegan fruit jams, chutneys, or preserves to complement the cheese flavors.

Dips or Spreads: Serve hummus, tapenade, or other vegan spreads for extra dipping options.

Garnishes: Sprinkle some fresh herbs like basil, rosemary, or thyme over the cheeses or around the board for added aroma and visual appeal.

Presentation: Arrange everything on a large serving board or platter, placing the cheeses, crackers, and accompaniments in an aesthetically pleasing manner. Leave some space between items for easy grabbing and dipping.

CHAPTER THREE

Salads and Dressings

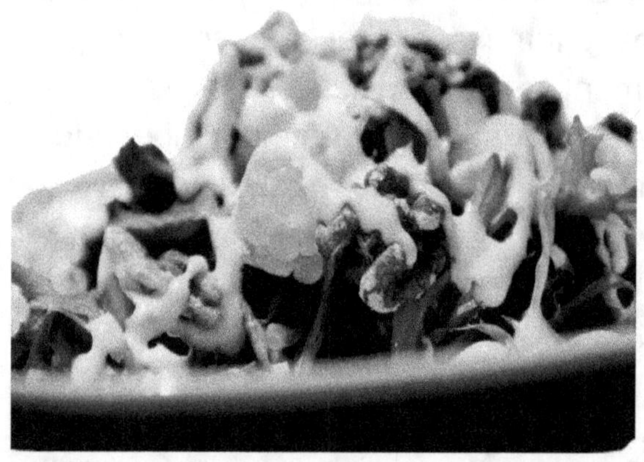

Salads on a vegetarian diet are versatile, nutritious, and can be customized to suit personal preferences. Here's an overview:

Base Ingredients: Start with a variety of fresh leafy greens like lettuce, spinach, kale, arugula, or mixed greens. These provide a nutrient-rich foundation for your salad.

Vegetables: Add a colorful array of chopped or sliced vegetables such as tomatoes, cucumbers, bell peppers, carrots, radishes, onions, broccoli, cauliflower, or avocado. These provide texture, flavor, and additional nutrients.

Protein: Incorporate vegetarian sources of protein such as chickpeas, black beans, kidney beans, tofu, tempeh, quinoa, or edamame. These add substance to the salad and help keep you feeling satisfied.

Fruits: For a touch of sweetness, include fruits like berries, apples, pears, grapes, or citrus segments. They add a burst of flavor and extra vitamins.

Nuts and Seeds: Sprinkle toasted nuts or seeds such as almonds, walnuts, pecans, pumpkin seeds, or sunflower seeds for added crunch, protein, and healthy fats.

Cheese: If you're a lacto-vegetarian, consider adding some crumbled feta, goat cheese, or shredded cheddar for a creamy and tangy element.

Crunch: Add texture with toppings like croutons, tortilla strips, or crispy chickpeas.

Dressings: Dressings can make or break a salad. Opt for vegetarian-friendly dressings made from ingredients like olive oil, balsamic vinegar, lemon juice, Dijon mustard, tahini, yogurt, honey (if not strictly vegan), herbs, and spices. Experiment with different flavor combinations like classic vinaigrettes, creamy tahini dressings, or Asian-inspired sesame ginger dressings.

When preparing salads on a vegetarian diet, the key is to include a balance of flavors, textures, and nutrients to create a satisfying and delicious meal or side dish. Feel free to get creative with your ingredient combinations and dressings to keep your salads exciting and enjoyable.

Quinoa and Roasted Vegetable Salad

A Quinoa and Roasted Vegetable Salad is a nutritious and flavorful dish that is perfect for a vegetarian diet. Here's an explanation of the ingredients and their health benefits:

Quinoa: Quinoa is a gluten-free whole grain that is high in protein, making it an excellent source of plant-based protein for vegetarians. It is also rich in fiber, providing digestive health benefits, and contains essential nutrients such as iron, magnesium, and manganese. Quinoa is a complete protein, meaning it contains all nine essential amino acids that the body cannot produce on its own.

Roasted Vegetables: Roasted vegetables like bell peppers, zucchini, eggplant, carrots, and onions add a delicious flavor and texture to the salad.

They are packed with vitamins, minerals, and antioxidants that support overall health. Roasting vegetables enhances their natural sweetness and caramelizes their sugars, making them even more delicious.

Leafy Greens: Adding leafy greens such as spinach, kale, or arugula to the salad provides additional fiber, vitamins (such as vitamin A, vitamin C, and vitamin K), and minerals (such as calcium and iron). Leafy greens are low in calories and high in antioxidants, which help reduce inflammation and protect against chronic diseases.

Herbs and Spices: Fresh herbs like parsley, cilantro, or basil, as well as spices like cumin, paprika, or garlic powder, can be used to season the salad and enhance its flavor without adding extra calories or sodium.

Healthy Fats: If you're making a salad, think about including nuts, seeds, or avocado slices as sources of healthy fats. These fats are necessary for proper food absorption, brain and heart health, and brain function. In instance, avocado offers potassium, fiber, and monounsaturated fats.

Dressing: Prepare a homemade dressing using heart-healthy oils like olive oil, along with vinegar or citrus juice, herbs, and spices. Avoid store-bought dressings that may be high in added sugars, sodium, and unhealthy fats.

Greek Salad with Tofu Feta

For those who are vegetarians, a tasty and nourishing option is a Greek salad with tofu feta. The components and their health advantages are explained as follows:

Tofu Feta: Made from soybeans, tofu is a well-liked plant-based protein source. With a comparable texture and flavor profile to genuine feta cheese, tofu feta is a dairy-free substitute. For vegans trying to obtain enough protein, tofu is a great choice because it is high in protein and low in calories. Tofu is also a good source of calcium, iron, and other important elements.

Fresh Vegetables: A Greek Salad typically includes fresh vegetables such as tomatoes, cucumbers, bell peppers, red onions, and olives. These vegetables are rich in vitamins, minerals, and antioxidants.

Tomatoes, for example, are a great source of vitamin C, potassium, and lycopene, a powerful antioxidant that may reduce the risk of chronic diseases.

Leafy Greens: Greek salads often feature leafy greens like romaine lettuce or mixed greens. Leafy greens are low in calories and high in fiber, vitamins, and minerals. They promote digestive health, support immune function, and may reduce the risk of heart disease and certain cancers.

Olives: An essential component of Greek cooking, olives give the salad a flavorful kick. Monounsaturated fats, which are heart-healthy fats that may help lower the risk of heart disease, are abundant in them. Antioxidants and anti-inflammatory substances can also be found in olives.

Herbs and Spices: Garlic and black pepper are used as well as herbs like mint and oregano to season Greek salads. These spices and herbs offer extra health advantages in addition to flavor. For instance, oregano has a high antioxidant content and potential antibacterial qualities.

Dressing: A basic dressing consisting of olive oil, red wine vinegar or lemon juice, garlic, and herbs is usually used for Greek salads. An essential part of the Mediterranean diet, olive oil is high in antioxidants and monounsaturated fats. It might lessen inflammation, raise cholesterol, and stave off heart disease.

Citrusy Kale Salad with Creamy Tahini Dressing

For those on a vegetarian diet, a citrusy kale salad with creamy tahini dressing is a tasty and nourishing choice. The components and their health advantages are explained as follows:

Kale: Kale is a nutrient-dense leafy green vegetable that is rich in vitamins, minerals, and antioxidants. It is particularly high in vitamin K, vitamin A, and vitamin C, as well as calcium and potassium. Kale is also a good source of fiber and may help reduce the risk of chronic diseases such as heart disease and certain types of cancer.

Citrus Fruits: Citrus fruits like oranges, grapefruits, or mandarins add a refreshing burst of flavor to the salad.

They are high in vitamin C, which boosts immune function and helps the body absorb iron from plant-based sources like kale. Citrus fruits also contain antioxidants and phytochemicals that may protect against inflammation and oxidative stress.

Avocado: Avocado offers fiber, healthy fats, and a creamy, rich taste to the salad. Because of their high content of monounsaturated fats, avocados may help lower bad cholesterol and the risk of heart disease. In addition, they include folate, potassium, and vitamin K, among other vital minerals.

Tahini Dressing: Tahini is a paste made from ground sesame seeds and is commonly used in Mediterranean and Middle Eastern cuisines. Tahini dressing is creamy and flavorful, and it adds a rich, nutty taste to the salad.

Tahini is a good source of healthy fats, protein, and minerals such as calcium, magnesium, and iron. It also contains antioxidants and may help reduce inflammation and improve heart health.

Additional Ingredients: You can customize your salad with other vegetarian-friendly ingredients such as cherry tomatoes, cucumber slices, shredded carrots, toasted nuts or seeds, and fresh herbs like parsley or cilantro. These ingredients add texture, flavor, and additional nutrients to the salad.

CHAPTER FOUR

Soups and Stews

Soups and stews are versatile and hearty options for those following a vegetarian diet. Here's an explanation of the ingredients and their benefits:

Vegetables: Vegetables are the star ingredients in vegetarian soups and stews. You can use a variety of fresh or frozen vegetables such as carrots, celery, onions, bell peppers, tomatoes, potatoes, squash, kale, spinach, peas, and mushrooms. Vegetables are rich in vitamins, minerals, fiber, and antioxidants, making them essential for overall health and well-being.

Legumes: Legumes like lentils, beans (such as black beans, kidney beans, chickpeas), and split peas are excellent sources of plant-based protein, fiber, and complex carbohydrates. They add texture, flavor, and nutritional value to soups and stews while helping to keep you feeling full and satisfied.

Grains: Grains such as rice, quinoa, barley, farro, or pasta can be added to soups and stews to provide additional bulk and nutrients. Whole grains are high in fiber, vitamins, and minerals, and they help regulate blood sugar levels and promote digestive health.

Broths and Stocks: A lot of vegetarian soups and stews start with a vegetable broth or stock. You can use homemade or store-bought broth, based on your desire. Stocks and broths give the food body and nutrition while contributing rich taste.

Herbs and Spices: Herbs and spices like garlic, ginger, thyme, rosemary, oregano, cumin, paprika, and chili powder enhance the flavor of vegetarian soups and stews without adding extra calories or sodium. They also provide additional health benefits, such as anti-inflammatory and antioxidant properties.

Healthy Fats: Vegetarian soups and stews can benefit from the subtle taste and texture boost that comes from a tiny addition of healthy fats like avocado, coconut milk, or olive oil. It takes healthy fats for hormone production, nutrient absorption, and brain function.

Toppings: Garnishes like fresh herbs, chopped green onions, grated cheese (if lacto-vegetarian), avocado slices, toasted nuts or seeds, or a dollop of yogurt or sour cream (if lacto-vegetarian) can add a finishing touch to vegetarian soups and stews, adding extra flavor and texture.

All things considered, soups and stews are wholesome, cozy dishes that work well with a vegetarian diet. They supply vital nutrients and support general health and wellbeing while providing a tasty way to include a range of veggies, legumes, grains, and spices in your meals.

Lentil and Vegetable Soup

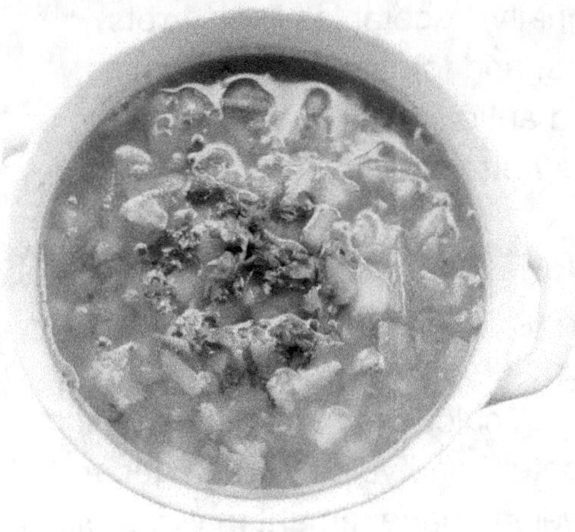

Lentil and vegetable soup is a nutritious and efficient option for a vegetarian diet for several reasons:

Protein Source: Lentils are a great source of plant-based protein, making them an essential component of a vegetarian diet. They provide a substantial amount of protein to help meet daily requirements.

Nutrient Dense: Lentils are rich in essential nutrients such as iron, folate, potassium, and fiber. Additionally, vegetables like carrots, celery, onions, and tomatoes add vitamins, minerals, and antioxidants to the soup, enhancing its nutritional value.

Minimal Calorie Content: The combination of low-calorie veggies and lentils provides a substantial and gratifying dinner without overindulging in calories, thanks to their high nutritional content and volume. Both general health and weight management may benefit from this.

Fiber Content: Lentils and vegetables are high in dietary fiber, which aids in digestion, helps maintain healthy cholesterol levels, and promotes satiety, keeping you feeling full for longer periods. This can be particularly beneficial for those following a vegetarian diet, as fiber helps meet the increased nutritional needs associated with plant-based eating.

Versatility: Lentil and vegetable soup can be easily customized based on personal preferences and ingredient availability. You can add a variety of vegetables, herbs, and spices to tailor the flavor to your liking, ensuring a diverse and enjoyable vegetarian meal.

Budget-Friendly: Lentils and vegetables are typically inexpensive and readily available, making lentil and vegetable soup a cost-effective option for individuals following a vegetarian diet. It allows for nutritious meals without breaking the bank.

Easy to Prepare: Lentil and vegetable soup is simple to prepare, requiring minimal cooking skills and time. It can be made in large batches and stored for later consumption, providing convenient and healthy meal options throughout the week.

Here's a simple recipe to prepare lentil and vegetable soup:

Ingredients:
1 cup dried lentils (any variety)
1 onion, diced
2 carrots, diced
2 celery stalks, diced
2 cloves garlic, minced
1 can (14 oz) diced tomatoes
6 cups vegetable broth
1 teaspoon dried thyme
1 teaspoon dried oregano
Salt and pepper to taste
Olive oil for cooking
Fresh parsley for garnish (optional)
Instructions:

Rinse Lentils: Start by rinsing the lentils under cold water in a fine-mesh strainer and set them aside.

Sauté Vegetables: Heat a large pot over medium heat and add a drizzle of olive oil. Add diced onion, carrots, and celery to the pot and cook for about 5 minutes, or until the vegetables begin to soften.

Add Garlic and Spices: Add minced garlic, dried thyme, and dried oregano to the pot, and cook for another minute until fragrant.

Combine Ingredients: Add the rinsed lentils, diced tomatoes (with their juices), and vegetable broth to the pot. Stir everything together.

Simmer: Bring the soup to a boil, then reduce the heat to low and let it simmer for about 25-30 minutes, or until the lentils are tender.

Add salt and pepper to taste when preparing the soup. As necessary, adjust the seasoning.

Serve: Once the lentils are cooked and the soup has thickened slightly, remove the pot from the heat. Ladle the soup into bowls and garnish with fresh parsley if desired.

Enjoy: Serve the lentil and vegetable soup hot and enjoy!

Feel free to customize the recipe by adding other vegetables such as spinach, kale, or potatoes, and adjust the seasonings to suit your taste preferences. This recipe is versatile and can easily be adapted based on what ingredients you have on hand.

Creamy Mushroom and Wild Rice Soup

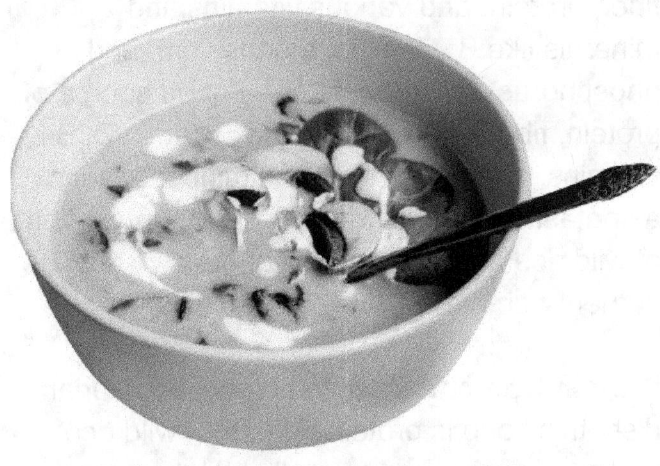

Creamy Mushroom and Wild Rice Soup is an efficient option for a vegetarian diet due to several reasons:

Nutritional Value: This soup is packed with nutrients essential for a balanced vegetarian diet. Wild rice provides complex carbohydrates, fiber, protein, and various vitamins and minerals like B vitamins, magnesium, and phosphorus. Mushrooms are a good source of protein, fiber, vitamins (such as vitamin D, B vitamins, and vitamin C), and minerals (such as potassium and selenium). The combination of wild rice and mushrooms offers a nutrient-rich meal.

Protein Content: Despite being a vegetarian dish, this soup is protein-rich. Both wild rice and mushrooms are naturally high in protein, making this soup a satisfying and nourishing option for vegetarians looking to meet their protein needs without relying on meat.

Satiety and Weight Management: The fiber content from wild rice and vegetables, along with the protein from mushrooms, helps promote satiety and keep you feeling full for longer periods. This can aid in weight management by reducing overall calorie intake and preventing overeating.

Creaminess without Dairy: The creaminess of this soup is achieved without using dairy cream, making it suitable for vegetarians who avoid dairy or for those following a vegan diet. The use of coconut cream or plant-based cream substitutes provides a creamy texture without compromising on flavor or richness.

Versatility and Customization: This soup is highly versatile and can be customized based on personal preferences and ingredient availability. You can add additional vegetables such as carrots, celery, or spinach for extra nutrients and flavor. You can also adjust the seasonings and herbs to suit your taste preferences.

Budget-Friendly: Wild rice and mushrooms are relatively affordable ingredients, making this soup a budget-friendly option for vegetarians. It allows individuals to enjoy a nutritious and flavorful meal without breaking the bank.

Ease of Preparation: Creamy Mushroom and Wild Rice Soup is simple to prepare and requires basic cooking skills. It can be made in a single pot, minimizing cleanup time. Additionally, leftovers can be stored and reheated for future meals, providing convenient and healthy options for busy schedules.

Overall, Creamy Mushroom and Wild Rice Soup is efficient for a vegetarian diet as it offers a nutrient-rich, protein-packed, and satisfying meal option that is both delicious and easy to prepare. It provides a balanced combination of carbohydrates, protein, fiber, vitamins, and minerals, making it a valuable addition to a vegetarian meal plan.

Here's a recipe for creamy mushroom and wild rice
soup:

Ingredients:
1 cup wild rice, uncooked
8 oz mushrooms, sliced (any variety you prefer)
1 onion, diced
3 cloves garlic, minced
4 cups vegetable broth
2 cups water
1 cup heavy cream (or substitute with coconut cream for a vegan option)
2 tablespoons all-purpose flour (or gluten-free flour)
2 tablespoons olive oil
1 teaspoon dried thyme
1 teaspoon dried rosemary
Salt and pepper to taste
Fresh parsley for garnish (optional).

Instructions:

Cook Wild Rice: Rinse the wild rice under cold water in a fine-mesh strainer. In a separate pot, cook the wild rice according to package instructions until tender. Drain any excess water and set aside.

Sauté Vegetables: Place a large saucepan over medium heat with olive oil. Add the sliced mushrooms and chopped onion to the pot. Cook for 5 to 7 minutes, or until the mushrooms are golden brown and the onions are transparent. When aromatic, add the minced garlic and simmer for one more minute.

Make Roux: To make a roux, sprinkle flour over the cooked vegetables and whisk to mix. Simmer for a minute or two to eliminate the taste of uncooked flour.

Add Broth and Water: Slowly pour in the vegetable broth and water, stirring constantly to prevent lumps from forming. Bring the mixture to a simmer.

Simmer: Fill the pot with cooked wild rice, dried thyme, and dried rosemary. Allow the soup to gently simmer for 15 to 20 minutes, so that the flavors can combine and the soup gets a little thicker.

Add Cream: Simmer for a further five minutes after stirring in the heavy cream (or coconut cream). To get the right consistency, you can add more broth or water if the soup is too thick.

Add salt and pepper to taste when preparing the soup. As necessary, adjust the seasoning.

Serve: Ladle the creamy mushroom and wild rice soup into bowls and garnish with fresh parsley if desired.

Enjoy: Serve the soup hot and enjoy the creamy, comforting flavors!

Feel free to customize the recipe by adding other vegetables such as carrots or celery, or by incorporating your favorite herbs and spices. This creamy mushroom and wild rice soup is hearty, satisfying, and perfect for chilly days.

Spicy Black Bean Chili

Spicy Black Bean Chili is an excellent choice for a vegetarian diet due to its nutritional profile, flavor, and versatility. Here's a comprehensive explanation of why it's efficient for vegetarians:

Protein Source: The main component of this chili, black beans, are an excellent plant-based source of protein. They are an essential part of a vegetarian diet since they supply a significant quantity of protein. For general health, muscle growth, and repair, protein is necessary.

Nutrient Dense: Black beans are not only rich in protein but also in fiber, vitamins, and minerals. They contain significant amounts of folate, iron, potassium, and magnesium, which are essential nutrients often lacking in vegetarian diets.

Additionally, other ingredients such as tomatoes, onions, and bell peppers contribute to the overall nutrient density of the chili.

Low in Saturated Fat: Unlike traditional meat-based chilis, Spicy Black Bean Chili is naturally low in saturated fat. This makes it a heart-healthy option for vegetarians, as diets high in saturated fat can increase the risk of heart disease and other health issues. Instead, the fats in this chili primarily come from heart-healthy sources like olive oil.

High in Fiber: Black beans are an excellent source of dietary fiber, which is beneficial for digestive health and can help prevent constipation. A high-fiber diet is also associated with a reduced risk of chronic diseases such as heart disease, diabetes, and certain types of cancer. Additionally, fiber helps promote satiety, making you feel fuller for longer periods and potentially aiding in weight management.

Antioxidant-Rich: Ingredients like tomatoes, onions, and bell peppers are rich in antioxidants, which help protect cells from damage caused by harmful molecules called free radicals. Consuming antioxidant-rich foods as part of a vegetarian diet may help reduce the risk of chronic diseases and support overall health and well-being.

Customizable: Spicy Black Bean Chili is highly customizable to suit individual taste preferences and dietary restrictions. You can adjust the level of spiciness by adding more or fewer chili peppers, and you can add additional vegetables such as corn, zucchini, or sweet potatoes for extra flavor and nutrients.

Easy to Prepare: This chili is relatively easy to prepare and can be made in large batches, making it perfect for meal prep or feeding a crowd. It requires minimal cooking skills and can be ready in under an hour, providing a convenient option for busy weeknights or lazy weekends.

Overall, Spicy Black Bean Chili is an efficient choice for a vegetarian diet because it offers a balanced combination of protein, fiber, vitamins, and minerals, while also being flavorful, satisfying, and easy to prepare. Incorporating this chili into a vegetarian meal plan can help ensure you're meeting your nutritional needs while enjoying delicious and nourishing meals.

CHAPTER FIVE

Main Courses

Main courses for a vegetarian diet encompass a wide range of delicious and nutritious options that are centered around plant-based ingredients. Here's a comprehensive explanation of main courses suitable for a vegetarian diet:

Plant-Based Proteins: Vegetarian main courses often feature plant-based proteins such as beans, lentils, tofu, tempeh, seitan, and chickpeas. These ingredients are versatile and can be used in various cuisines and cooking methods to create satisfying and protein-rich dishes.

Whole Grains: Whole grains like quinoa, brown rice, barley, farro, bulgur, and whole wheat pasta are staples in vegetarian cooking. They provide complex carbohydrates, fiber, and essential nutrients, serving as a hearty base for many main dishes.

Vegetables: Vegetables play a crucial role in vegetarian main courses, providing flavor, texture, and a wide array of vitamins, minerals, and antioxidants. From leafy greens and cruciferous vegetables to root vegetables and nightshades, there's a vast selection to choose from to create diverse and nutritious meals.

Nuts and Seeds: Nuts and seeds add crunch, flavor, and nutritional value to vegetarian main courses. They can be used as toppings, garnishes, or incorporated into dishes to provide healthy fats, protein, and micronutrients. Examples include almonds, walnuts, pumpkin seeds, sunflower seeds, and sesame seeds.

Dairy and Plant-Based Alternatives: Dairy products such as cheese, yogurt, and milk are common ingredients in vegetarian cooking, providing richness and creaminess to dishes. For those following a vegan diet or avoiding dairy, there are plenty of plant-based alternatives made from soy, almonds, coconut, oats, and other sources.

Eggs: Eggs are a versatile ingredient in vegetarian cooking, providing protein and nutrients. They can be used to make omelets, frittatas, quiches, and egg-based dishes like scrambled eggs or shakshuka.

Herbs and Spices: Herbs and spices are essential for adding flavor and depth to vegetarian main courses. From aromatic herbs like basil, cilantro, and parsley to spices like cumin, paprika, turmeric, and chili powder, there's a wide range of seasonings to enhance the taste of vegetarian dishes.

Cuisine Variety: Vegetarian main courses can draw inspiration from various cuisines around the world, including Mediterranean, Asian, Indian, Mexican, Middle Eastern, and more. Each cuisine offers unique flavors, ingredients, and cooking techniques that can be adapted to create delicious and satisfying vegetarian meals.

Overall, vegetarian main courses are diverse, flavorful, and nutritious, offering a plethora of options for individuals following a plant-based diet. By incorporating a variety of plant-based proteins, whole grains, vegetables, nuts, seeds, dairy or plant-based alternatives, eggs, herbs, and spices, you can create satisfying and balanced meals that cater to your taste preferences and dietary needs.

Eggplant Parmesan

Eggplant Parmesan is a classic Italian dish that's not only delicious but also an excellent choice for a vegetarian diet. Here's why it's a great option:

Nutrient-Rich: Eggplant is the star ingredient of Eggplant Parmesan, providing essential nutrients such as fiber, vitamins (including vitamin C, vitamin K, and vitamin B6), minerals (such as potassium and magnesium), and antioxidants. These nutrients support overall health and well-being, making Eggplant Parmesan a nutritious main course option for vegetarians.

Low in Calories: Eggplant is naturally low in calories and contains no fat or cholesterol, making it a healthy choice for those looking to manage their weight or improve their overall diet quality.

By baking the eggplant instead of frying it, you can further reduce the calorie content while still retaining its delicious flavor and texture.

Protein Source: While eggplant itself is not particularly high in protein, Eggplant Parmesan typically includes layers of cheese, such as mozzarella and Parmesan, which provide protein and add richness to the dish. Additionally, you can boost the protein content by incorporating a layer of vegetarian-friendly protein sources such as tofu or a plant-based meat substitute.

Versatility: Eggplant Parmesan is a versatile dish that can be adapted to suit individual taste preferences and dietary restrictions. You can customize the recipe by adding extra vegetables like spinach or mushrooms, or by adjusting the seasonings and herbs to create your own unique flavor profile. You can also make it gluten-free by using gluten-free breadcrumbs or flour.

Comfort Food Appeal: Eggplant Parmesan is a hearty and comforting dish that's perfect for satisfying cravings and providing a sense of indulgence without the need for meat. The layers of tender eggplant, gooey cheese, and flavorful marinara sauce create a mouthwatering combination that's sure to please vegetarians and meat-eaters alike.

Easy to Prepare: While Eggplant Parmesan may seem elaborate, it's actually quite simple to prepare. The basic steps involve slicing the eggplant, breading and baking the slices until golden and tender, layering them with marinara sauce and cheese, and baking until bubbly and melted. With just a few ingredients and minimal prep work, you can create a delicious and satisfying meal in no time.

Family-Friendly: Eggplant Parmesan is a crowd-pleaser that's perfect for serving to family and friends, whether they're vegetarian or not. It's comforting flavors and satisfying texture make it a favorite for gatherings, potlucks, and weeknight dinners alike.

Overall, Eggplant Parmesan is an excellent choice for a vegetarian diet due to its nutrient-rich ingredients, versatility, comfort food appeal, and ease of preparation. Whether you're looking for a satisfying meatless meal or simply want to switch up your dinner routine, Eggplant Parmesan is sure to become a new favorite in your recipe repertoire.

Chickpea Tikka Masala

Chickpea Tikka Masala is a flavorful and nutritious vegetarian dish that's perfect for those following a plant-based diet. Here's why it's a great option:

Protein-Rich: Chickpeas, also known as garbanzo beans, are the primary protein source in Chickpea Tikka Masala. They're packed with protein, making them a filling and satisfying option for vegetarians. Additionally, chickpeas are high in fiber, which aids in digestion and helps keep you feeling full longer.

Nutrient-Dense: Chickpeas are not only rich in protein but also in essential nutrients such as folate, iron, manganese, and phosphorus. These nutrients are important for overall health and well-being, making Chickpea Tikka Masala a nutritious addition to a vegetarian diet.

Flavorful Spices: Tikka Masala is known for its aromatic blend of spices, which gives the dish its signature flavor. Common spices used in Chickpea Tikka Masala include cumin, coriander, turmeric, paprika, and garam masala. These spices not only add depth and complexity to the dish but also provide additional health benefits due to their antioxidant and anti-inflammatory properties.

Versatility: Chickpea Tikka Masala is a versatile dish that can be customized to suit individual preferences. You can adjust the level of spiciness by adding more or fewer chili peppers, and you can add extra vegetables such as spinach, bell peppers, or cauliflower for added flavor and nutrients. You can also customize the sauce to your liking by adjusting the amount of coconut milk, tomato sauce, or yogurt used.

Dairy-Free Option: Traditional Tikka Masala recipes often include dairy products such as yogurt or cream. However, Chickpea Tikka Masala can easily be made dairy-free by using coconut milk or a plant-based yogurt alternative. This makes it suitable for vegans or those avoiding dairy products.

Easy to Prepare: Despite its complex flavors, Chickpea Tikka Masala is relatively easy to prepare. It involves sautéing onions, garlic, and spices, adding chickpeas and tomato sauce, and simmering until the flavors meld together. Serve it over rice or with naan bread for a complete and satisfying meal.

Satisfying and Comforting: Chickpea Tikka Masala is a comforting and hearty dish that's perfect for warming up on chilly evenings. Its rich and creamy sauce, paired with tender chickpeas and fragrant spices, makes it a satisfying option for vegetarians and meat-eaters alike.

Here's a simple recipe to prepare Chickpea Tikka Masala:

Two tablespoons of oil (vegetable or coconut oil) are the ingredients.
One finely chopped onion, three minced garlic cloves, and one inch of grated ginger
One can of 14 ounces of rinsed and drained chickpeas
One can, or fourteen ounces chopped tomatoes
One can, or fourteen ounces milk from coconuts
Two tablespoons tomato paste
One spoonful of masala gram
One-teaspoon each of ground coriander and cumin
half a teaspoon of turmeric powder
Half a teaspoon of paprika
Add salt and pepper to taste. Garnish with fresh cilantro, if desired.
Naan bread or cooked rice ready to be served.

Guidelines:
Heat oil in a big skillet or pot over medium heat to sauté aromatics. Add the chopped onion and simmer for about 5 minutes, or until softened. Cook for an additional one to two minutes, or until aromatic, after adding the grated ginger and minced garlic.

Add the Spices: Add the paprika, ground cumin, ground coriander, ground turmeric, and ground garam masala. Stirring continually, cook for 1 minute or until the spices become fragrant and roasted.

Add Tomato Paste and Diced Tomatoes: Stir together the tomato paste and diced tomatoes in the skillet. Simmer the mixture for five to seven minutes to let the flavors combine and the sauce gradually thicken.

Add Chickpeas: Add the drained and rinsed chickpeas to the skillet, stirring to coat them in the sauce. Let the mixture simmer for another 5 minutes to allow the flavors to combine.

Pour in Coconut Milk: Pour in the coconut milk, stirring to combine. Bring the mixture to a simmer and let it cook for an additional 10-15 minutes, stirring occasionally, until the sauce thickens and the chickpeas are heated through.

Season to Taste: Use salt and pepper to taste the sauce and adjust the seasoning as necessary. At this point, you can add a small sprinkle of cayenne pepper or chili powder if you want your food hotter.

Serve: Once the sauce has reached your desired consistency and the chickpeas are heated through, remove the skillet from the heat. Serve the Chickpea Tikka Masala hot over cooked rice or with naan bread, garnished with fresh cilantro if desired.

Enjoy: Serve immediately and enjoy the flavorful and comforting Chickpea Tikka Masala!

Feel free to customize the recipe by adding extra vegetables such as bell peppers, spinach, or cauliflower, or by adjusting the spices to suit your taste preferences. This versatile dish is sure to become a favorite in your vegetarian recipe repertoire.

Portobello Mushroom Steaks with Chimichurri Sauce

For a satisfying vegetarian dish packed with flavor, try Portobello Mushroom Steaks with Chimichurri Sauce. Here's a simple recipe to elevate your vegetarian diet:

Ingredients:
4 large Portobello mushrooms, stems removed
1/4 cup olive oil
2 tablespoons balsamic vinegar
3 cloves garlic, minced
Salt and pepper to taste
Chimichurri Sauce:
1 cup fresh parsley, chopped
1/4 cup fresh cilantro, chopped
3 cloves garlic, minced
1 shallot, finely chopped
1/4 cup red wine vinegar
1/2 cup olive oil
Salt and pepper to taste.

Instructions:
Set the temperature of your grill pan or grill to medium-high.

Mix the olive oil, balsamic vinegar, minced garlic, salt, and pepper in a small bowl. Apply the mixture on the Portobello mushrooms' two sides.

Place the mushrooms on the grill and cook for 4-5 minutes per side, or until they are tender and juicy.

While the mushrooms are grilling, prepare the chimichurri sauce. In a blender or food processor, combine parsley, cilantro, minced garlic, shallot, red wine vinegar, olive oil, salt, and pepper. Blend until smooth.

Once the mushrooms are cooked, remove them from the grill and let them rest for a few minutes.

To serve, spoon chimichurri sauce over the grilled Portobello mushroom steaks. Serve with your favorite sides such as roasted vegetables, quinoa, or a salad.

Enjoy these flavorful Portobello Mushroom Steaks with Chimichurri Sauce as a delicious and satisfying option for your vegetarian diet!

Portobello Mushroom Steaks with Chimichurri Sauce offer several health benefits:

Nutrient-Rich Mushrooms: Portobello mushrooms are low in calories but high in essential nutrients like fiber, vitamins, and minerals. They are a good source of B vitamins, potassium, and selenium, which support various bodily functions including metabolism and immune health.

Plant-Based Protein: Mushrooms are one of the few plant-based sources of complete protein, meaning they contain all nine essential amino acids our bodies need for muscle growth, repair, and overall health. This makes them an excellent option for vegetarians looking to increase their protein intake.

Heart Health: The olive oil used in both the marinade and chimichurri sauce is rich in monounsaturated fats, which are heart-healthy fats associated with reduced risk of cardiovascular diseases. Additionally, garlic, a key ingredient in both the marinade and sauce, has been linked to improved heart health by helping to lower cholesterol and blood pressure levels.

Antioxidants: The parsley, cilantro, and garlic in the chimichurri sauce are rich in antioxidants, which help protect cells from damage caused by free radicals and oxidative stress.

These compounds have anti-inflammatory properties and may reduce the risk of chronic diseases like cancer and heart disease.

Digestive Health: The fiber content of Portobello mushrooms and the fresh herbs in the chimichurri sauce support digestive health by promoting regularity, preventing constipation, and feeding beneficial gut bacteria.

CHAPTER SIX

Side Dishes

The following are thorough descriptions of side dishes that go well with a vegetarian diet:

Roasted veggies: Roasting veggies intensifies their flavors and brings forth their inherent sweetness. Vegetables like carrots, bell peppers, zucchini, broccoli, cauliflower, and cherry tomatoes can all be used.
Toss the veggies in olive oil, add salt, pepper, and your preferred herbs or spices (such as thyme, garlic powder, or rosemary) to season them, then roast them in the oven until they become soft and caramelized.

Quinoa salad: A wonderful complement to a vegetarian diet, quinoa is a nutrient-dense whole grain that is high in fiber and protein. It tastes great with crunchy veggies, fresh herbs, and a zesty vinaigrette.

As directed on the package, prepare the quinoa and allow it to cool. Add diced cucumbers, tomatoes, red onions, bell peppers, and fresh herbs (parsley, cilantro, etc.) along with a dressing (olive oil, lemon juice, garlic, salt, and pepper) after that.

Sweet Potato Wedges:

Sweet potatoes are rich in vitamins, minerals, and fiber, making them a nutritious choice for a side dish. Cutting them into wedges and roasting them in the oven creates a crispy exterior and a tender interior.

Toss sweet potato wedges in olive oil, season with salt, pepper, and your favorite spices (such as paprika or cumin), and roast until golden brown and cooked through.

Mediterranean Chickpea Salad: A variety of vegetarian dishes can be prepared with chickpeas, which are a highly adaptable legume. They give this salad taste and minerals, and fresh veggies and herbs contribute protein and fiber.

Add chopped cucumbers, cherry tomatoes, red onions, Kalamata olives, and crumbled feta cheese to the cooked chickpeas. Add olive oil, lemon juice, dried oregano, minced garlic, salt, and pepper to the salad.

Grilled asparagus: Low in calories but abundant in vitamins A, C, and K, fiber, and folate, asparagus is a nutrient-dense vegetable. Grilling adds a smoky flavor and brings out its inherent sweetness.

Arrange asparagus spears in an olive oil-tossing dish, add salt & pepper to taste, and grill until soft and gently browned. For added brightness, squeeze fresh lemon juice over the grilled asparagus just before serving.

Spinach and Feta Stuffed Mushrooms:
This side dish combines nutrient-rich spinach,
tangy feta cheese, and earthy mushrooms for a
flavorful and satisfying appetizer or
accompaniment.
To prepare, remove the stems from large
mushrooms and brush them with olive oil.
Sauté chopped spinach, garlic, and onions until
wilted, then mixed in crumbled feta cheese.
Stuff the mushroom caps with the spinach and
feta mixture, sprinkle with breadcrumbs, and
bake until the mushrooms are tender and the
filling is golden brown.

Cauliflower Rice Pilaf:
Cauliflower rice is a low-carb alternative to
traditional rice, making it suitable for various
dietary preferences. In this pilaf, cauliflower
rice is cooked with aromatic spices,
vegetables, and nuts for a flavorful and
nutritious side dish.

Sauté cauliflower rice with diced onions, carrots, peas, and your choice of nuts (such as almonds or cashews) in olive oil. Season with turmeric, cumin, coriander, and cinnamon for a fragrant pilaf. Finish with chopped fresh herbs like parsley or cilantro for added freshness.

Caprese salad: Made with fresh tomatoes, mozzarella cheese, basil, and balsamic glaze, this dish is a typical Italian meal. It highlights the flavors of ripe tomatoes and creamy mozzarella and is light and pleasant.
Arrange fresh mozzarella cheese and juicy tomato slices on a dish. Place a few fresh basil leaves in between the cheese and tomato pieces. Add a drizzle of extra virgin olive oil and balsamic glaze, then season with salt and pepper. Serve as a bright and light appetizer or side dish.

Grilled Vegetable Skewers: A colorful and delectable touch to any vegetarian dinner are grilled vegetable skewers. You can quickly bake them in the oven or on the barbecue, and they may be customized with your favorite vegetables.

Vegetable chunks such as red onions, bell peppers, cherry tomatoes, zucchini, and mushrooms should be woven onto skewers. Add your preferred herbs or spices, salt, and pepper to the skewers after brushing them with olive oil. Serve the vegetables as a vibrant and wholesome side dish after grilling or roasting them until they are soft and slightly browned.

Cucumber Avocado Salad:

This refreshing salad features crisp cucumber, creamy avocado, and tangy lime dressing for a burst of flavor and texture. It's light, hydrating, and pairs well with various main dishes.

Slice cucumbers and avocados and arrange them on a platter.

Drizzle with a dressing made from lime juice, olive oil, minced garlic, honey (or agave syrup for a vegan option), salt, and pepper. Garnish with chopped cilantro or mint for a refreshing twist.

These side dishes offer a diverse range of flavors, textures, and nutrients to complement your vegetarian meals and make them more satisfying and enjoyable.

Garlic and Herb Roasted Potatoes

Garlic and Herb Roasted Potatoes are a delightful and comforting side dish that pairs perfectly with any vegetarian meal. Here's how to make them:

Ingredients:
2 pounds potatoes (such as Yukon Gold or Russet), washed and cut into bite-sized cubes
3 tablespoons olive oil
4 cloves garlic, minced
1 teaspoon dried thyme
1 teaspoon dried rosemary
1 teaspoon dried oregano
Salt and pepper to taste
Chopped fresh parsley for garnish (optional)

Instructions:
To make cleanup easier, line a baking sheet with foil or parchment paper and preheat your oven to 425°F (220°C).

Toss the potato cubes until they are uniformly coated in a large bowl with olive oil, chopped garlic, dried thyme, dried rosemary, dried oregano, salt, and pepper.

Arrange the seasoned potatoes on the prepared baking sheet in a single layer, taking care not to pile them too closely together. This makes it possible for them to roast evenly and get a crispy outside.

Bake the potatoes for 25 to 30 minutes in a preheated oven, turning them over halfway through, or until the outside is crispy and golden brown and the center is still soft.

After the potatoes are perfectly roasted, take them out of the oven and place them on a platter for serving. Add some chopped fresh parsley as a garnish for some color and freshness.

Serve the Garlic and Herb Roasted Potatoes hot alongside your favorite vegetarian main dish, such as grilled vegetables, veggie burgers, or lentil stew.

Enjoy these flavorful and aromatic roasted potatoes as a satisfying and versatile side dish that will elevate your vegetarian meals!

Garlic and Herb Roasted Potatoes offer several health benefits, making them a nutritious addition to a vegetarian diet:

Rich in Potassium: Potatoes are a good source of potassium, an essential mineral that plays a crucial role in maintaining healthy blood pressure levels. Adequate potassium intake can help counteract the effects of sodium and reduce the risk of hypertension and cardiovascular diseases.

High in Vitamin C: Potatoes contain vitamin C, a powerful antioxidant that supports immune function, promotes skin health, and aids in wound healing. Garlic, another key ingredient in this dish, also provides vitamin C, along with other beneficial compounds that have antimicrobial properties.

Good Source of Fiber: Dietary fiber, which is crucial for digestive health, is found in both potatoes and garlic. Fiber promotes the growth of good gut flora, eases constipation, and helps control bowel motions. Consuming a high-fiber diet may also reduce the chance of getting chronic illnesses including colorectal cancer and several digestive issues.

Antioxidant Properties: Garlic contains sulfur compounds like allicin, which have antioxidant properties that help neutralize free radicals and reduce oxidative stress in the body. Antioxidants play a protective role against chronic diseases such as cancer, heart disease, and neurodegenerative disorders.

Heart Health: Olive oil, used in the roasting process, is rich in monounsaturated fats, which are associated with improved heart health. These healthy fats help lower LDL (bad) cholesterol levels and reduce the risk of coronary artery disease and stroke. Additionally, the herbs used in the seasoning, such as thyme, rosemary, and oregano, contain compounds that may support cardiovascular health and reduce inflammation.

Nutrient Density: Potatoes offer a number of important vitamins and minerals in a nutrient-dense food that is low in calories. You can add flavor to the dish without drastically raising the calorie or sodium load by adding garlic and herbs.

All things considered, Roasted Garlic and Herb Potatoes provide a tasty approach to take advantage of the health advantages of potatoes, garlic, olive oil, and herbs. This recipe, when made with healthy ingredients and consumed in moderation, can help provide a vegetarian diet that is both balanced and nutrient-dense.

Lemon Asparagus with Almonds

This colorful and nourishing side dish of lemon asparagus with almonds goes well with a vegetarian diet. This is how to make this tasty dish:

Ingredients:
1 bunch asparagus, tough ends trimmed
2 tablespoons olive oil
2 cloves garlic, minced
Zest of 1 lemon
Juice of 1/2 lemon
1/4 cup sliced almonds
Salt and pepper to taste
Fresh parsley for garnish (optional).

Guidelines:
Get the asparagus ready: After washing, cut off the tough ends of the asparagus spears. You can use a knife to cut them or break off the woody ends to accomplish this. Using paper towels, pat dry the asparagus.

Sauté the Garlic and Almonds: In a large skillet, heat the olive oil over medium heat. Add the minced garlic and sliced almonds to the skillet and sauté for 1-2 minutes, stirring frequently, until the almonds are lightly toasted and the garlic is fragrant.

To cook the asparagus, place the trimmed spears in a skillet with the almonds and garlic. Sauté the asparagus for five to seven minutes, stirring now and again, until it's soft but still crunchy. Depending on the asparagus stalks' thickness, the cooking time can change.

Add Lemon Zest and Juice: Once the asparagus is cooked to your desired tenderness, add the lemon zest and juice to the skillet. Stir to coat the asparagus evenly with the lemony flavor. The lemon zest adds brightness, while the lemon juice adds a refreshing tang.

Season and Serve: Season the lemon asparagus with salt and pepper to taste. Transfer the cooked asparagus to a serving platter, garnish with fresh parsley if desired, and serve immediately.

Lemon Asparagus with Almonds offers numerous health benefits, making it an excellent addition to a vegetarian diet:

Nutrient-Rich Asparagus: Asparagus is packed with essential vitamins and minerals, including vitamins A, C, E, and K, as well as folate, iron, and potassium. These nutrients support various bodily functions such as immune health, bone health, and blood clotting.

Antioxidant Properties: Asparagus contains antioxidants like vitamin C and glutathione, which help neutralize harmful free radicals in the body and reduce oxidative stress. By protecting cells from damage, antioxidants may lower the risk of chronic diseases like cancer, heart disease, and neurodegenerative disorders.

Heart Health: Asparagus is low in calories and fat but high in fiber and folate, all of which are beneficial for heart health. Fiber helps lower cholesterol levels and improve digestion, while folate helps regulate homocysteine levels in the blood, reducing the risk of heart disease.

Healthy Fats from Almonds: Almonds are a rich source of monounsaturated fats, which are heart-healthy fats associated with reduced risk of cardiovascular disease. They also contain vitamin E, magnesium, and antioxidants, all of which contribute to heart health by reducing inflammation and improving cholesterol levels.

Bone Health: Asparagus is a good source of vitamin K, which plays a crucial role in bone health by aiding in calcium absorption and promoting bone mineralization. Adequate intake of vitamin K may help reduce the risk of osteoporosis and fractures.

Digestive Health: The fiber content in asparagus supports digestive health by promoting regularity, preventing constipation, and feeding beneficial gut bacteria. Additionally, almonds contain both soluble and insoluble fiber, which can improve digestive function and help maintain a healthy weight.

Immune Support: The vitamin C found in both asparagus and lemon juice boosts immune function by supporting the production of white blood cells and enhancing the body's ability to fight infections. A strong immune system is essential for overall health and well-being.

Coconut Curried Cauliflower

Coconut Curried Cauliflower is a flavorful and nutritious dish suitable for a vegetarian diet. Here's a comprehensive explanation:

Ingredients:
Cauliflower: Provides fiber, vitamins, and minerals.
Coconut milk: Adds creaminess and richness to the dish.
Curry powder: Infuses the dish with aromatic spices like turmeric, coriander, cumin, and chili.
Vegetables: You can add veggies like bell peppers, peas, or carrots for added texture and nutrition.
Garlic and ginger: Enhance flavor and add depth to the curry.
Onion: Adds sweetness and depth to the sauce.

Add salt and pepper to taste and season the dish.
Optional garnishes include chopped nuts, fresh cilantro, or a squeeze of lime.

Instructions:
Preheat the oil in a big saucepan or skillet over medium heat.
Stir in the ginger, garlic, and onion. Sauté until aromatic and mellow.
To toast the spices, stir in the curry powder and simmer for an additional minute.
When the cauliflower florets start to soften, add them to the skillet and simmer.
Add the coconut milk and mix everything together. Simmer the mixture for a while.
When the cauliflower is soft, heat it covered, stirring now and then.
If you want to add more veggies, add them to the curry and simmer them until they are soft.

To taste, add salt and pepper for seasoning.
Serve the Coconut Curried Cauliflower hot,
topped with chopped almonds, fresh cilantro,
or, if preferred, a squeeze of lime juice.

Benefits to nutrition: Cauliflower is high in
antioxidants, fiber, and vitamins C and K.
Without using dairy, coconut milk adds
smoothness and healthy fats.
Curry powder contains spices that have
anti-inflammatory qualities, such as turmeric.
Vegetables add more fiber, vitamins, and
minerals to the dish.

CHAPTER SEVEN

Pasta and Grain Dishes

Pasta and grain dishes are versatile and satisfying options for vegetarians, providing a range of nutrients and flavors. Here's an overview:

Pasta Dishes:
Vegetable Primavera: A colorful pasta dish loaded with seasonal vegetables like bell peppers, zucchini, cherry tomatoes, and broccoli, tossed in olive oil, garlic, and herbs. Spinach and Ricotta Stuffed Shells: Jumbo pasta shells filled with a creamy mixture of spinach, ricotta cheese, garlic, and herbs, baked in marinara sauce.

Pesto Pasta: Pasta coated in a vibrant basil pesto sauce made with fresh basil leaves, pine nuts, garlic, Parmesan cheese (or nutritional yeast for vegans), and olive oil.
Creamy Mushroom Pasta: Linguine or fettuccine tossed in a creamy sauce made with sautéed mushrooms, garlic, thyme, and a splash of cream or plant-based milk.
Spaghetti Aglio e Olio: A simple yet flavorful dish featuring spaghetti tossed in garlic-infused olive oil, red pepper flakes, parsley, and a squeeze of lemon juice.

Grain Dishes:
Quinoa Salad: Nutrient-packed quinoa mixed with diced cucumbers, tomatoes, bell peppers, red onion, and fresh herbs, dressed with lemon vinaigrette.
Vegetable Fried Rice: Brown rice stir-fried with an assortment of vegetables like carrots, peas, bell peppers, and green onions, seasoned with soy sauce and sesame oil.

Mushroom Risotto: Creamy Arborio rice cooked with sautéed mushrooms, shallots, garlic, white wine, and vegetable broth, finished with butter (or olive oil for vegans) and Parmesan cheese (or nutritional yeast for vegans).

Mexican Quinoa Casserole: Layers of cooked quinoa, black beans, corn, bell peppers, onions, salsa, and cheese (or vegan cheese) baked until bubbly and golden.

Tabbouleh: A refreshing Middle Eastern salad made with bulgur wheat, chopped parsley, tomatoes, cucumbers, red onion, lemon juice, and olive oil.

When preparing pasta and grain dishes on a vegetarian diet, you can easily incorporate protein sources like beans, tofu, tempeh, or plant-based meat substitutes to ensure a balanced meal. Additionally, don't forget to experiment with different herbs, spices, and sauces to add variety and depth to your dishes. Enjoy the endless possibilities of vegetarian pasta and grain creations!

here's a general guide on how to prepare a simple yet delicious vegetable primavera pasta dish:

**Vegetable Primavera Pasta
Ingredients:**
8 ounces of your favorite pasta (spaghetti, fettuccine, or penne)
2 tablespoons olive oil
3 cloves garlic, minced
1 medium onion, thinly sliced
2 cups assorted vegetables (bell peppers, zucchini, cherry tomatoes, broccoli, etc.), chopped
Salt and pepper to taste
1/4 cup fresh basil leaves, chopped (optional)
Grated Parmesan cheese or nutritional yeast (optional).

Instructions:
Cook the Pasta:
Heat a big saucepan of salted water till it boils.
When the pasta is al dente, add it and cook it
as directed on the package.
After the pasta has cooked, drain it and set it
aside, saving about 1/2 cup of the pasta water.

Sauté the Vegetables: In a large skillet set
over medium heat, warm up the olive oil while
the pasta cooks.
To the skillet, add the thinly sliced onion and
minced garlic. Sauté the onion for two to three
minutes, or until it is aromatic and transparent.
Include the chopped veggies in the skillet.
Cook the vegetables for 5 to 7 minutes, stirring
occasionally, or until they are crisp but still soft.
To taste, add salt and pepper to the
vegetables. Add chopped basil leaves, if using,
and stir.

Mix Pasta and veggies: Put the cooked pasta
and the sautéed veggies in a skillet.
Mix everything together so that the flavors of
the vegetables seep into the pasta.
To create a light sauce, add a splash of the
pasta water that was set aside if the pasta
appears dry.

Serve: Take the skillet off the burner as soon
as everything is thoroughly heated and mixed.
Use salt and pepper to season food according
to taste.
For extra taste, you can also top the spaghetti
with nutritional yeast or grated Parmesan
cheese before serving.
If preferred, garnish with extra finely chopped
basil leaves.
Enjoy your veggie primavera pasta hot out of
the pot!

Spinach and Ricotta Stuffed Shells

Here's a guide on how to prepare Spinach and Ricotta Stuffed Shells, a delightful vegetarian dish:

Ingredients:
1 box (12 ounces) jumbo pasta shells
2 cups ricotta cheese
1 cup chopped spinach, cooked and drained
1 cup shredded mozzarella cheese
1/2 cup grated Parmesan cheese
2 cloves garlic, minced
1 egg, lightly beaten
1 teaspoon dried oregano
1 teaspoon dried basil
Salt and pepper to taste
2 cups marinara sauce
Fresh basil leaves for garnish (optional).

Instructions:
Preheat the Oven:
Preheat your oven to 350°F (175°C).
Cook the Pasta Shells:

Heat a big saucepan of salted water till it boils.
As directed on the package, cook the giant
pasta shells until they are al dente.
To end the cooking process, drain the shells
and give them a quick rinse under cold water.
Put aside.

Prepare the Filling:
In a large mixing bowl, combine the ricotta
cheese, chopped spinach, shredded
mozzarella cheese, grated Parmesan cheese,
minced garlic, beaten egg, dried oregano, dried
basil, salt, and pepper. Mix until well combined.

Stuff the Shells:
Spoon the ricotta and spinach mixture into
each cooked pasta shell until they are full but
not overstuffed.

Put the Plate Together:
Line the bottom of a baking dish with a thin
layer of marinara sauce.
Place the filled shells in a single layer in the
baking dish.
Evenly top the packed shells with the
remaining marinara sauce.

Bake: Place aluminum foil over the baking dish
and bake in the preheated oven for 25 to 30
minutes, or until the sauce is bubbling and the
shells are thoroughly warm.

Serve: After baking, take off the foil and give
the dish a few minutes to cool before cutting
into portions.
If desired, garnish with fresh basil leaves.
Enjoy the hot spinach and ricotta stuffed shells!

This dish is a comforting and satisfying option for vegetarians, packed with creamy ricotta cheese, nutritious spinach, and flavorful herbs. It's perfect for a family dinner or a gathering with friends. Feel free to customize the recipe by adding other vegetables or herbs to the filling, or by using your favorite marinara sauce. Buon !

Spinach and Ricotta Stuffed Shells offer numerous health benefits, particularly when prepared with wholesome ingredients and balanced portions:

Rich in Protein: Ricotta cheese is a significant source of protein, providing essential amino acids necessary for muscle repair, immune function, and overall health. This makes the dish a satisfying and filling option, especially for vegetarians who may need to ensure they're getting enough protein in their diet.

Packed with Nutrients: Spinach is a nutrient powerhouse, containing vitamins A, C, and K, as well as folate, iron, and magnesium. These nutrients support various bodily functions, including immune health, bone health, and blood clotting.

Calcium Content: Ricotta and Parmesan cheeses contribute to the dish's calcium content, essential for maintaining strong bones and teeth. This is particularly beneficial for vegetarians who may have limited sources of dietary calcium.

Fiber from Vegetables: Spinach adds dietary fiber to the dish, aiding digestion, promoting satiety, and supporting heart health. Fiber also helps regulate blood sugar levels and may reduce the risk of certain chronic diseases, such as diabetes and heart disease.

Low in Saturated Fat: When prepared with moderation and using low-fat cheese options, Spinach and Ricotta Stuffed Shells can be a relatively low-saturated fat dish. This supports heart health by helping to maintain healthy cholesterol levels and reducing the risk of cardiovascular disease.

Antioxidant Properties: Spinach contains antioxidants such as vitamin C and beta-carotene, which help protect cells from damage caused by free radicals. These antioxidants play a role in reducing inflammation and lowering the risk of chronic diseases, including cancer and heart disease.

Vegetarian-Friendly: As a vegetarian dish, Spinach and Ricotta Stuffed Shells provide an alternative source of protein and nutrients for individuals following a plant-based diet. By incorporating a variety of vegetables and dairy products, it offers a well-rounded meal option that meets nutritional needs.

Versatility and Customization: This dish can be easily customized to include additional vegetables, herbs, or whole-grain pasta for added fiber and nutrients. By experimenting with different ingredients, individuals can tailor the dish to their taste preferences and dietary requirements.

Overall, Spinach and Ricotta Stuffed Shells offer a delicious way to incorporate nutrient-dense ingredients into a vegetarian diet, promoting overall health and well-being. Enjoying this dish as part of a balanced diet can contribute to a nutritious and satisfying meal option.

Vegetable Stir-Fry with Soba Noodles

Here's a detailed explanation of how to prepare Vegetable Stir-Fry with Soba Noodles, a delicious and nutritious vegetarian dish:

Ingredients:
Soba Noodles: Soba noodles are thin Japanese noodles made from buckwheat flour, which adds a nutty flavor and a hearty texture to the dish. You'll need about 8 ounces of soba noodles.

Assorted Vegetables: Choose a variety of colorful vegetables for your stir-fry, such as bell peppers, broccoli, carrots, snap peas, mushrooms, and onions. Aim for about 4 cups of chopped vegetables in total.

Sauce Ingredients:

Soy Sauce: Use about 1/4 cup of soy sauce as the base for your stir-fry sauce. You can use low-sodium soy sauce if preferred.

Rice Vinegar: Add 2 tablespoons of rice vinegar for acidity and tanginess.

Sesame Oil: Use 1 tablespoon of sesame oil to add depth of flavor and aroma.

Garlic and Ginger: Mince 2 cloves of garlic and 1 tablespoon of fresh ginger to infuse the sauce with savory and aromatic notes.

Sriracha or Chili Garlic Sauce (optional): For a spicy kick, add 1-2 teaspoons of Sriracha or chili garlic sauce.

Honey or Brown Sugar (optional): Add sweetness to balance the flavors, using 1-2 teaspoons of honey or brown sugar.

Garnish (optional):

Green Onions: Thinly slice green onions to sprinkle on top of the finished dish.
Sesame Seeds: Toasted sesame seeds add crunch and nuttiness as a garnish.

Guidelines:
Prepare Soba Noodles:
Heat up a big saucepan of water until it boils. Add the soba noodles and simmer for the recommended amount of time (typically 4-5 minutes), or until al dente, per the instructions on the package.
To halt the cooking process, drain the cooked noodles and give them a quick rinse under cold water. Put them away.

Prepare Stir-Fry Sauce:
In a small bowl, whisk together soy sauce, rice vinegar, sesame oil, minced garlic, minced ginger, Sriracha or chili garlic sauce (if using), and honey or brown sugar (if using). Set the sauce aside.

Stir-Fry Vegetables: In a big skillet or wok, heat up one tablespoon of oil over medium-high heat.

Cook the chopped veggies in the skillet for two to three minutes, starting with the tougher ones like broccoli and carrots.

When the vegetables are crisp-tender, add softer veggies such bell peppers, snap peas, mushrooms, and onions and simmer for an additional two to three minutes.

After making the stir-fry sauce, pour it over the veggies and toss to coat them thoroughly.

Simmer the sauce for a further one to two minutes, or until it slightly thickens.

Mix with Soba Noodles: Include the stir-fried vegetables in a skillet with the cooked soba noodles.

Mix everything until the noodles are well heated and covered with sauce.

Serve: Take the skillet off the burner as soon as everything is thoroughly heated and mixed. Distribute the Soba Noodle and Vegetable Stir-Fry among serving dishes.
If preferred, garnish with toasted sesame seeds and sliced green onions.
Enjoy your tasty and nourishing vegetarian dinner while it's still hot!

Health Benefits:
Nutrient-Rich Vegetables: This dish is loaded with a variety of colorful vegetables, providing essential vitamins, minerals, and antioxidants for overall health and well-being.
High in Fiber: Soba noodles and vegetables contribute dietary fiber, promoting digestion, satiety, and heart health.

Protein: Although this dish is vegetarian, you can add protein sources like tofu, tempeh, or edamame to increase its protein content and make it more satisfying.

Low in Saturated Fat: When prepared with minimal oil and a balanced sauce, this dish is relatively low in saturated fat, supporting heart health.

Customizable: You can customize this dish with your favorite vegetables, adjust the level of spiciness, and tailor the sauce to your taste preferences.

Quick and Easy: Vegetable Stir-Fry with Soba Noodles is a quick and easy meal option, perfect for busy weeknights or when you're short on time.

Overall, this dish offers a flavorful, satisfying, and nutritious option for vegetarians, packed with wholesome ingredients and vibrant flavors. Enjoy experimenting with different vegetables and flavors to create your perfect stir-fry!

Creamy Pumpkin Risotto

Creamy Pumpkin Risotto is a delicious and comforting dish perfect for vegetarians, especially during the fall season when pumpkins are abundant. Here's how to prepare it:

Ingredients:
Arborio Rice: Arborio rice is the preferred rice for risotto due to its high starch content, which creates a creamy texture. You'll need about 1 ½ cups of Arborio rice for this recipe.

Pumpkin Puree: Use about 1 cup of pumpkin puree made from roasted or steamed pumpkin. You can also use canned pumpkin puree for convenience.

Vegetable Broth: Approximately 4-5 cups of vegetable broth will be needed to cook the risotto. Use low-sodium broth if available.

Onion and Garlic: Finely chop 1 onion and mince 2 cloves of garlic to add flavor to the risotto.

Butter (or Olive Oil): Use about 2 tablespoons of butter or olive oil for sautéing the onion and garlic and adding richness to the risotto.

Parmesan Cheese (or Nutritional Yeast): Grate about ½ cup of Parmesan cheese to add a savory flavor and creaminess to the risotto. For a vegan option, substitute with nutritional yeast.

White Wine (optional): Adding about ½ cup of dry white wine enhances the flavor of the risotto, but it can be omitted if preferred.

Pumpkin Pie Spice (optional): For extra warmth and flavor, you can add a teaspoon of pumpkin pie spice or a combination of cinnamon, nutmeg, ginger, and cloves.

Salt and Pepper: To taste, for seasoning the risotto.

Guidelines:
Get the pumpkin puree ready. If you're using fresh pumpkin, roast or steam it until it becomes soft, then puree it in a food processor or blender until it's smooth. Skip this step if you're using canned pumpkin puree.

Warm the Vegetable Broth: Place the vegetable broth in a saucepan and heat it over medium-low heat until it becomes warm. Throughout the cooking process, keep it warm.

Sauté the onion and garlic: Melt the butter (or heat the olive oil) in a large skillet or Dutch oven over medium heat. Saute the minced garlic and finely diced onion for two to three minutes, or until the ingredients are fragrant and tender.

Toast the Rice: Combine the Arborio rice, onion, and garlic in a pan. Once the rice is lightly browned and covered with butter (or oil), stir and cook for an additional one to two minutes.

Deglaze with Wine (optional): Pour in the white wine (if using) and stir, allowing the rice to absorb the wine. Cook until the wine has mostly evaporated, stirring occasionally.

Add Pumpkin Puree: Stir in the pumpkin puree until well combined with the rice mixture.

To begin cooking the risotto, add a ladleful of the heated vegetable stock to the skillet at a time while stirring continuously. Before adding more broth, let the rice absorb it. Al dente rice is creamy and tender but yet slightly firm to the bite. Continue cooking while stirring periodically. Usually, this takes between 18 and 20 minutes.

Finish and Season: Add salt, pepper, and pumpkin pie spice (if using) to the risotto once it reaches the right consistency, tasting as you go. Add the nutritional yeast or grated Parmesan cheese and stir until it melts and becomes creamy.

To serve, distribute the smooth and creamy pumpkin risotto onto bowls or serving plates. If preferred, garnish with more grated Parmesan cheese. Enjoy it while it's hot!

Health Benefits:
Nutrient-Rich Pumpkin: Pumpkin is rich in vitamins A, C, and E, as well as fiber and antioxidants. It supports immune function, eye health, and overall well-being.

Whole Grain Rice: Arborio rice used in risotto retains more nutrients compared to refined rice varieties. It provides complex carbohydrates for sustained energy and dietary fiber for digestive health.

Vegetarian-Friendly: This dish is entirely vegetarian, making it suitable for individuals following a plant-based diet.
Customizable: You can customize this risotto by adding additional vegetables like spinach or mushrooms for extra nutrition and flavor.

Warm and Comforting: Creamy pumpkin risotto is a comforting and satisfying meal option, perfect for chilly autumn evenings. Enjoy this creamy pumpkin risotto as a flavorful and nutritious addition to your vegetarian diet!

CHAPTER EIGHT

Breads and Baked Goods

Breads and baked goods play a significant role in a vegetarian diet, providing essential carbohydrates, fiber, and sometimes protein. Here's a comprehensive explanation of various types of breads and baked goods suitable for a vegetarian diet:

Whole Grain Breads: Made from whole grains, which maintain their bran, germ, and endosperm, whole grain breads include whole wheat, oat, and multigrain varieties. They are abundant in antioxidants, vitamins, minerals, and fiber.
Because whole grain breads contain complex carbs, they are suitable for vegetarians and offer long-lasting energy.
Toasted and paired with hummus, avocado, or nut butter, they make a satisfying and healthy lunch or snack.

Artisan Breads:

Artisan breads are typically made with simple ingredients like flour, water, salt, and yeast or sourdough starter. They come in various shapes, sizes, and flavors, often featuring crusty exteriors and chewy interiors.

Common types include baguettes, ciabatta, sourdough, and focaccia.

Artisan breads are versatile and can be enjoyed on their own, dipped in olive oil and balsamic vinegar, or used as a base for sandwiches and bruschetta.

Flatbreads:

Flatbreads are thin, unleavened breads that can be made from various grains, including wheat, corn, or chickpea flour.

Examples include naan, pita, tortillas, and lavash.

Flatbreads are commonly used to wrap sandwiches, as a base for pizzas, or served alongside dips and spreads like hummus or tzatziki.

Savory Baked Goods:
Savory baked goods like savory muffins,
scones, or biscuits can be made with
ingredients like cheese, herbs, vegetables, and
spices.
They are perfect for breakfast, brunch, or as a
side dish for soups and salads.
Veggie-packed options include spinach and
feta muffins, roasted vegetable scones, or
sun-dried tomato and basil biscuits.

Sweet Baked Goods:
Sweet baked goods include a wide range of
treats like muffins, cakes, cookies, and
pastries.
Vegetarian-friendly options often incorporate
fruits, nuts, seeds, and spices for added flavor
and nutrition.
Examples include banana bread, zucchini
muffins, apple cinnamon scones, and pumpkin
spice cookies.

Specialty Breads:

Specialty breads encompass a variety of breads made with unique ingredients or techniques, such as gluten-free breads, seed breads, or sprouted grain breads.

They cater to specific dietary preferences or restrictions and can be enjoyed by vegetarians seeking alternative options.

Homemade Breads:

Making bread at home allows for full control over ingredients and customization to suit dietary preferences.

Home-baked breads can be made with whole grains, seeds, nuts, and dried fruits for added nutrition and flavor.

Additionally, homemade bread-making can be a rewarding and therapeutic activity, providing a sense of accomplishment and satisfaction.

Whole Wheat Olive Bread

Whole Wheat Olive Bread is a flavorful and nutritious bread that combines the earthy taste of whole wheat flour with the briny richness of olives. Here's a comprehensive explanation:

Ingredients:
Whole Wheat Flour: The base of the bread, providing fiber, vitamins, minerals, and antioxidants. Whole wheat flour retains the bran and germ of the wheat kernel, offering more nutrients compared to refined white flour.

Olives: Pitted and chopped olives add a savory and tangy flavor to the bread. Choose your favorite variety, such as Kalamata, black, or green olives, for added depth of flavor.

Yeast: Yeast is the leavening agent that gives bread its light, fluffy texture and causes it to rise. You can use quick yeast or active dry yeast.

Olive Oil: Adds richness and moisture to the bread, enhancing its texture and flavor. Olive oil also contributes heart-healthy monounsaturated fats.

Salt: Enhances the flavor of the bread and helps regulate yeast activity.

Optional Ingredients: You can customize your Whole Wheat Olive Bread by adding ingredients like fresh herbs (rosemary or thyme), garlic, sun-dried tomatoes, or cheese for extra flavor and variety.

Instructions:

Activate the Yeast: In a small bowl, dissolve the yeast in warm water according to the package instructions. Let it sit for a few minutes until frothy, indicating that the yeast is active.

Mix the Dough: Put the whole wheat flour, chopped olives, olive oil, and salt in a sizable mixing bowl. Add the combination of activated yeast and stir until a rough dough forms.

Knead the dough: Place the dough on a surface dusted with flour and work it for 8 to 10 minutes, or until it is smooth and elastic. To keep it from sticking, add extra flour as needed.

First Rise: Put the dough in a bowl that has been lightly oiled, cover it with a fresh kitchen towel or plastic wrap, and let it rise for one to two hours, or until it has doubled in size, in a warm, draft-free environment.

Shape the Bread: Punch down the dough to get rid of any air bubbles once it has risen. Form it into an oval or round loaf and transfer it to a baking pan covered with parchment paper.

Second Rise: Cover the shaped loaf with a towel and let it rise for another 30-45 minutes, or until it puffs up slightly.

Preheat the Oven: While the bread is rising, preheat your oven to 375°F (190°C).

Bake the Bread: Once the bread has risen, slash the top with a sharp knife to allow for expansion during baking. Bake in the preheated oven for 30-35 minutes, or until the crust is golden brown and the bread sounds hollow when tapped on the bottom.

Cool and Serve: Transfer the baked bread to a wire rack and let it cool completely before slicing. Enjoy your Whole Wheat Olive Bread sliced and served with butter, olive oil, or your favorite toppings.

Nutritional Benefits:
Whole Wheat Flour: Provides fiber, vitamins B and E, minerals such as magnesium and iron, and antioxidants that support digestive health, heart health, and overall well-being.

Olives: Rich in monounsaturated fats, antioxidants, and anti-inflammatory compounds. Olives may help lower cholesterol levels, reduce inflammation, and protect against chronic diseases.

Olive Oil: Contains heart-healthy monounsaturated fats, antioxidants, and anti-inflammatory properties. Olive oil may support cardiovascular health, reduce inflammation, and improve cholesterol levels.

Customizable: You can customize Whole Wheat Olive Bread with additional ingredients like herbs, garlic, or sun-dried tomatoes for added flavor and nutrition.

Whole Wheat Olive Bread is a delicious and nutritious addition to a vegetarian diet, offering a balance of whole grains, healthy fats, and savory flavors. Enjoy it as a wholesome accompaniment to soups, salads, or as a satisfying snack on its own.

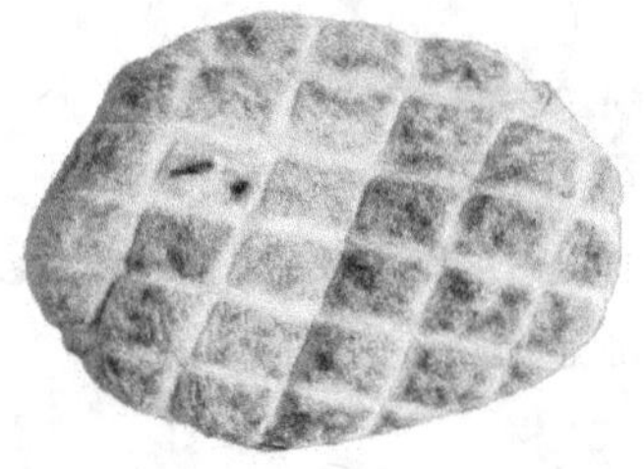

Vegan Banana Nut Muffins

Vegan Banana Nut Muffins are a delicious and wholesome treat suitable for a vegetarian diet. Here's a comprehensive explanation of how to prepare them:

Ingredients:
Bananas: Ripe bananas serve as the primary sweetener and binder in vegan banana nut muffins. Use mashed bananas to add moisture and natural sweetness to the muffins.

Flour: Choose all-purpose flour or whole wheat flour as the base for the muffins. Whole wheat flour adds fiber and nutrients, while all-purpose flour yields a lighter texture.

Plant-Based Milk: Use your favorite plant-based milk, such as almond milk, soy milk, or oat milk, to moisten the batter and create a tender crumb. Unsweetened varieties are recommended to control the sweetness of the muffins.

Neutral Oil: A neutral-flavored oil like vegetable oil or melted coconut oil helps keep the muffins moist. Avoid using strong-flavored oils like olive oil, as they may overpower the delicate banana flavor.

Maple Syrup or Agave Nectar: Natural liquid sweeteners like maple syrup or agave nectar add sweetness and complexity to the muffins without the need for refined sugar.

Vanilla Extract: Vanilla extract enhances the flavor of the muffins, adding warmth and depth.

Baking Powder and Baking Soda: These leavening agents help the muffins rise and achieve a light and fluffy texture.

Salt: A pinch of salt balances the sweetness and enhances the flavors of the muffins.

Chopped Nuts: Walnuts or pecans add a crunchy texture and nutty flavor to the muffins. Chop them finely for even distribution throughout the batter.

Instructions:
Preheat the Oven: Preheat your oven to 350°F (175°C) and line a muffin tin with paper liners or grease the cavities with oil or cooking spray.

Prepare the Wet Ingredients: In a mixing bowl, mash the ripe bananas with a fork until smooth. Add the plant-based milk, neutral oil, maple syrup or agave nectar, and vanilla extract. Mix until well combined.

Combine the Dry Ingredients: In a separate mixing bowl, whisk together the flour, baking powder, baking soda, and salt.

Pour the wet ingredients into the bowl containing the dry ingredients to combine the batter. Take care not to overmix; stir just until incorporated. Once the chopped nuts are equally incorporated into the batter, fold them in.

Fill the Muffin Cups: Using a spoon or cookie scoop, fill each muffin cup about two-thirds full with the batter.

Bake the Muffins: Place the muffin tin in the preheated oven and bake for 20-25 minutes, or until the muffins are golden brown and a toothpick inserted into the center comes out clean.

Cool and Serve: Remove the muffin tin from the oven and let the muffins cool in the pan for 5 minutes before transferring them to a wire rack to cool completely. Enjoy your vegan banana nut muffins warm or at room temperature.

Nutritional Benefits:
Bananas: Rich in potassium, fiber, and vitamins B6 and C. Bananas provide natural sweetness and moisture to the muffins without the need for added sugar.

Whole Wheat Flour: Adds fiber, vitamins, minerals, and antioxidants to the muffins, supporting digestive health and overall well-being.

Nuts: Provide healthy fats, protein, fiber, vitamins, and minerals. Nuts contribute to heart health, satiety, and balanced nutrition.

Plant-Based Ingredients: Vegan banana nut muffins are free from animal products, making them suitable for individuals following a vegetarian or vegan diet. They offer a compassionate and sustainable alternative to traditional muffin recipes.

Vegan banana nut muffins are a nutritious and satisfying snack or breakfast option, perfect for vegetarians looking for a wholesome treat. Enjoy them as a grab-and-go snack or pair them with a hot cup of coffee or tea for a delightful morning indulgence.

Rosemary Garlic Focaccia

Rosemary Garlic Focaccia is a delightful and flavorful bread that's perfect for vegetarians. Here's a comprehensive explanation of how to prepare it:

Ingredients:
All-Purpose Flour: Provides the base for the focaccia dough, giving it structure and texture. You'll need about 3 to 4 cups of all-purpose flour.

Yeast: Works as a leavening agent to give the dough a light, fluffy texture and to cause it to rise. You can use quick yeast or active dry yeast.

Water: Hydrates the dough and activates the yeast.

Olive Oil: Adds richness and moisture to the focaccia, enhancing its flavor and texture. Some olive oil is also used for greasing the pan and drizzling over the top of the bread.

Salt: Enhances the flavor of the bread and helps regulate yeast activity.

Rosemary: Fresh rosemary sprigs or dried rosemary add a fragrant and aromatic flavor to the focaccia. Rosemary pairs wonderfully with garlic and olive oil, contributing to the classic flavor profile of this bread.

Garlic: Fresh garlic cloves, minced or thinly sliced, infuse the focaccia with a robust garlic flavor when baked.

Coarse Salt: Sprinkled over the top of the focaccia before baking, coarse salt adds a crunchy texture and enhances the savory flavors of the bread.

Instructions:

Activate the Yeast: In a small bowl, dissolve the yeast in warm water according to the package instructions. Let it sit for a few minutes until frothy, indicating that the yeast is active.

To prepare the dough, place the flour, olive oil, salt, and activated yeast mixture in a large mixing bowl. Stir to produce a rough dough.

Knead the dough: Place the dough on a surface dusted with flour and work it for 8 to 10 minutes, or until it is smooth and elastic. To keep it from sticking, add extra flour as needed.

First Rise: Put the dough in a bowl that has been lightly oiled, cover it with a fresh kitchen towel or plastic wrap, and let it rise for one to two hours, or until it has doubled in size, in a warm, draft-free environment.

Shape the Focaccia: Once the dough has risen, punch it down to release any air bubbles. Transfer it to a lightly greased baking sheet or pan and gently press it into an even layer, spreading it out to fill the pan.

Second Rise: Cover the shaped focaccia dough with a towel and let it rise for another 30-45 minutes, or until it puffs up slightly.

Preheat the Oven: While the dough is rising, preheat your oven to 425°F (220°C).

Top the Focaccia: Using your fingers or the handle of a wooden spoon, make indentations all over the surface of the risen dough. Drizzle olive oil over the top and sprinkle minced garlic and fresh rosemary leaves. Sprinkle coarse salt evenly over the top.

Bake the Focaccia: Place the focaccia in the preheated oven and bake for 20-25 minutes, or until golden brown and crispy on the edges.

Cool and Serve: Remove the focaccia from the oven and let it cool slightly before slicing and serving. Enjoy your rosemary garlic focaccia warm or at room temperature.

Nutritional Benefits:
All-Purpose Flour: Provides carbohydrates for energy and small amounts of protein. While not as nutrient-dense as whole grain flours, it serves as the base for the focaccia dough.

Olive Oil: Rich in heart-healthy monounsaturated fats and antioxidants, olive oil adds richness and moisture to the focaccia. It also contributes to the savory flavor profile of the bread.

Rosemary: Aromatic and flavorful, rosemary adds a burst of freshness to the focaccia. It contains antioxidants and anti-inflammatory compounds, offering potential health benefits.

Garlic: Besides enhancing the flavor of the focaccia, garlic is known for its immune-boosting properties and potential cardiovascular benefits.

Coarse Salt: While used sparingly, coarse salt adds flavor and texture to the focaccia. It also helps balance the sweetness of the bread and enhances its savory notes.

Rosemary Garlic Focaccia is a delicious and aromatic bread that's perfect for serving as an appetizer, accompaniment to a meal, or as a standalone snack. Its savory flavors and soft, chewy texture make it a crowd-pleaser among vegetarians and non-vegetarians alike. Enjoy it fresh from the oven or toasted with a drizzle of olive oil for a delightful culinary experience.

CHAPTER NINE

Desserts

Desserts for a vegetarian diet encompass a wide range of sweet treats that exclude meat and fish products but may include dairy, eggs, and other animal-derived ingredients. Here's a comprehensive explanation of various dessert options suitable for a vegetarian diet:

1. **Fruit-Based Desserts:**
Fruit-based desserts utilize fresh, canned, or dried fruits as the main ingredient. Examples include fruit salads, fruit parfaits, fruit crisps, fruit tarts, and fruit sorbets.
These desserts are naturally sweet and refreshing, providing vitamins, minerals, fiber, and antioxidants essential for overall health.

They can be enjoyed as a light and guilt-free dessert option or dressed up with toppings like whipped cream, yogurt, nuts, or chocolate for added indulgence.

2. **Baked Goods:**

Baked goods encompass a wide variety of sweet treats made from flour, sugar, eggs, and other ingredients. Vegetarian-friendly options include cakes, cupcakes, cookies, brownies, muffins, scones, and pastries.

Baked goods can be customized with various flavors, fillings, and toppings to suit personal preferences and dietary needs.

Alternative ingredients like plant-based milk, flaxseed meal, and applesauce can be used to veganize traditional recipes, making them suitable for vegetarians and vegans alike.

3. **Dairy-Based Desserts:**

Dairy-based desserts include a range of creamy and indulgent treats made with milk, cream, yogurt, cheese, and other dairy products. Examples include ice cream, pudding, custard, cheesecake, panna cotta, and tiramisu.

Vegetarians who consume dairy products can enjoy these desserts for their rich and creamy texture, as well as their diverse flavors and varieties.

Opt for high-quality, organic dairy products whenever possible to support animal welfare and environmental sustainability.

4. **Chocolate and Confections:**

Chocolate and confections offer a decadent and indulgent option for dessert lovers. Vegetarian-friendly choices include chocolate bars, truffles, fudge, chocolate-covered fruits or nuts, and candies.

Look for chocolate products labeled as "vegetarian" or "dairy-free" to ensure they do not contain animal-derived ingredients like gelatin or milk powder.
Dark chocolate, in particular, is a rich source of antioxidants and may offer health benefits when consumed in moderation.

5. **Frozen Desserts:**
Frozen desserts provide a cool and refreshing option, especially during hot weather. Vegetarian-friendly choices include ice cream, gelato, sorbet, frozen yogurt, and popsicles. Look for dairy-free or vegan options made with plant-based milk alternatives like almond, coconut, or soy milk for a cruelty-free and dairy-free treat.
Experiment with different flavors, mix-ins, and toppings to create customized frozen desserts that cater to individual tastes and preferences.

6. **Specialty Desserts:**

Specialty desserts encompass a variety of unique and exotic treats from around the world. Examples include Indian sweets like gulab jamun and jalebi, Middle Eastern desserts like baklava and , and Asian desserts like mochi and mango sticky rice.

Many specialty desserts can be adapted to suit a vegetarian diet by omitting or substituting non-vegetarian ingredients.

These desserts offer an opportunity to explore different cultures and culinary traditions while satisfying sweet cravings.

Nutritional Considerations:

While desserts are often considered indulgent treats, they can still be part of a balanced and nutritious diet when enjoyed in moderation.

Opt for desserts made with whole food ingredients like fruits, nuts, whole grains, and natural sweeteners for added nutritional value.

Consider portion sizes and balance sweet treats with healthier choices to maintain overall dietary balance and support optimal health.

Vegan Chocolate Avocado Mousse

Vegan Chocolate Avocado Mousse is a creamy and decadent dessert that's perfect for vegetarians looking for a dairy-free and egg-free option. Here's a comprehensive explanation of this delicious treat:

Ingredients:

Avocado: Ripe avocados serve as the base for this mousse, providing a creamy texture and healthy fats. Avocados are rich in monounsaturated fats, fiber, vitamins, and minerals.

Cocoa Powder: Unsweetened cocoa powder adds rich chocolate flavor to the mousse without the need for dairy chocolate. Choose high-quality cocoa powder for the best taste.

Sweetener: The mousse is sweetened with natural sweeteners such as dates, agave nectar, or maple syrup. Depending on how sweet you desire, adjust the amount.

Plant-Based Milk: Plant-based milk, such as almond milk, coconut milk, or soy milk, helps thin out the mousse and achieve the desired consistency. Use unsweetened and unflavored milk for the best results.

Vanilla Extract: Vanilla extract enhances the flavor of the mousse, adding warmth and depth.

Optional Ingredients: You can customize your Vegan Chocolate Avocado Mousse with additional ingredients like nut butter (such as almond or peanut butter), vanilla bean paste, or spices (such as cinnamon or chili powder) for added flavor complexity.

Instructions:
Prepare the Avocados: Scoop the flesh of ripe
avocados into a blender or food processor,
discarding the pits and skins.

Add Ingredients: Add cocoa powder,
sweetener, plant-based milk, and vanilla
extract to the blender or food processor.

Blend Until Smooth: Blend the ingredients
until smooth and creamy, scraping down the
sides of the blender or food processor as
needed to ensure everything is well combined.

Adjust Consistency: If the mousse is too
thick, you can add a little more plant-based
milk to thin it out to your desired consistency.
Blend again until smooth.

Taste and Adjust: Taste the mousse and adjust the sweetness or flavorings as needed. Add more sweetener, cocoa powder, or vanilla extract to suit your preferences.

Chill: Transfer the mousse to a bowl or individual serving dishes and refrigerate for at least 30 minutes to allow it to chill and set slightly.

Serve: Once chilled, remove the mousse from the refrigerator and serve it topped with fresh berries, sliced fruit, chopped nuts, or coconut whipped cream, if desired.

Storage: Store any leftover mousse in an airtight container in the refrigerator for up to 2-3 days.

Nutritional Benefits:

Avocado: Provides healthy monounsaturated fats, fiber, vitamins (such as vitamin E, vitamin K, and vitamin C), and minerals (such as potassium and magnesium). Avocado promotes heart health, satiety, and glowing skin.

Cocoa Powder: Rich in antioxidants, flavonoids, and minerals (such as iron and magnesium), cocoa powder offers potential health benefits, including improved mood, cognitive function, and heart health.

Natural Sweeteners: Maple syrup, agave nectar, or dates provide sweetness without refined sugar, offering a healthier alternative while still satisfying sweet cravings.

Plant-Based Milk: Offers calcium, vitamin D, and protein, while being lactose-free and cholesterol-free. Plant-based milk supports bone health, muscle growth, and overall well-being.

Vegan Chocolate Avocado Mousse is a delicious and nutritious dessert option for vegetarians seeking a dairy-free and egg-free treat. Its creamy texture and rich chocolate flavor make it a crowd-pleaser for any occasion. Enjoy this guilt-free indulgence knowing that it's made with wholesome ingredients and packed with beneficial nutrients.

Berry Crisp with Oatmeal Pecan Topping

Berry Crisp with Oatmeal Pecan Topping is a delightful and comforting dessert that's perfect for vegetarians. Here's a comprehensive explanation:

Ingredients:

Berries: Choose your favorite berries or a mix of berries such as strawberries, blueberries, raspberries, and blackberries. Berries provide natural sweetness, fiber, vitamins, and antioxidants.

Sugar: Sweetens the berry filling and enhances the natural flavors of the berries. You can use granulated sugar, brown sugar, or alternative sweeteners like maple syrup or honey.

Cornstarch: Helps thicken the berry filling by absorbing excess liquid during baking.

Lemon Juice: Adds brightness and balances the sweetness of the berries. Lemon juice also helps prevent the berries from oxidizing and turning brown.

Vanilla Extract: Enhances the flavor of the berry filling with a hint of warmth and sweetness.

Old-Fashioned Rolled Oats: The base of the crisp topping, providing texture and nutty flavor. Rolled oats are a good source of fiber, vitamins, and minerals.

Flour: Binds the crisp topping ingredients together and helps create a crumbly texture. All-purpose flour or whole wheat flour can be used.

Brown Sugar: Sweetens the crisp topping and adds a caramel-like flavor. You can also use granulated sugar or coconut sugar as alternatives.

Pecans: Chopped pecans give the topping a richness and crunch. Pecans are an excellent source of antioxidants, protein, and beneficial fats.

Cinnamon: Adds warmth and depth of flavor to the crisp topping. You can also add other spices like nutmeg or cardamom for additional complexity.

Salt: Balances the sweetness and enhances the flavors of the crisp topping.

Butter (or Vegan Butter): Adds richness and helps bind the topping ingredients together. Use unsalted butter or vegan butter for vegetarians or vegans.

Instructions:

Prepare the Berry Filling: In a large mixing bowl, combine the berries, sugar, cornstarch, lemon juice, and vanilla extract. Toss until the berries are evenly coated, then transfer the mixture to a baking dish.

To make the Crisp Topping, place the flour, brown sugar, chopped pecans, cinnamon, and salt in a separate mixing bowl. Mix thoroughly to mix in all the ingredients. Next, add the butter, cut into small pieces, and use your fingers or a pastry cutter to work it into the dry ingredients until the mixture resembles coarse crumbs.

Assemble the Crisp: Sprinkle the crisp topping evenly over the berry filling in the baking dish, covering the berries completely.

Bake: Place the baking dish in a preheated oven and bake the berry crisp at 375°F (190°C) for 35-40 minutes, or until the topping is golden brown and the berry filling is bubbly.

To serve, take the berry crisp out of the oven and allow it to cool down a little. If preferred, top warm servings with a dollop of whipped cream or a scoop of vanilla ice cream.

Storage: You may keep any leftover berry crisp in the fridge for two to three days. Before serving, reheat in the microwave or oven.

Nutritional Benefits:
Berries: Rich in vitamins, minerals, fiber, and antioxidants, berries offer numerous health benefits, including improved heart health, cognitive function, and immune support.

Oats: Provide complex carbohydrates, fiber, protein, and various nutrients like iron, magnesium, and zinc. Oats support digestive health, satiety, and blood sugar control.

Pecans: High in healthy fats, protein, fiber, vitamins, and minerals, pecans promote heart health, brain function, and overall well-being.

Natural Sweeteners: When used in moderation, natural sweeteners like sugar, maple syrup, or honey offer a better alternative to refined sugar, providing sweetness without the added chemicals or empty calories.
Berry Crisp with Oatmeal Pecan Topping is a delicious and wholesome dessert option for vegetarians, offering a balance of sweet and tart flavors, crisp and crunchy textures, and nourishing ingredients. Enjoy it as a comforting treat on its own or as a delightful ending to any meal.

Coconut Mango Sorbet

Coconut Mango Sorbet is a refreshing and tropical dessert perfect for vegetarians. Here's a comprehensive explanation:

Ingredients:

Mangoes: Ripe mangoes are the star ingredient of this sorbet, providing natural sweetness, vibrant color, and a tropical flavor. Mangoes are rich in vitamins A and C, fiber, and antioxidants.

Coconut Milk: Creamy coconut milk adds richness and a hint of coconut flavor to the sorbet. Opt for full-fat coconut milk for the creamiest texture, but light coconut milk can also be used for a lighter option.

Sugar: Sweetens the sorbet and balances the tartness of the mangoes. You can use granulated sugar, coconut sugar, or alternative sweeteners like agave nectar or maple syrup.

Lime Juice: Adds brightness and acidity to the sorbet, enhancing the flavor of the mangoes. Lime juice also helps prevent the sorbet from becoming too sweet and adds a refreshing zing.

Optional Ingredients: You can customize your Coconut Mango Sorbet with additional ingredients like shredded coconut, fresh mint leaves, or a splash of rum for added flavor complexity.

Instructions:

Prepare the Mangoes: Peel and dice the ripe mangoes, discarding the pits. For a smoother texture, you can puree the mango flesh in a blender or food processor until smooth.

Mix the Ingredients: In a mixing bowl, combine the pureed mangoes, coconut milk, sugar, and lime juice. Stir until the sugar is dissolved and the mixture is well combined.

Taste and Adjust: Taste the sorbet mixture and adjust the sweetness or tartness as needed by adding more sugar or lime juice.

Chill the Mixture: Cover the bowl with plastic wrap or a lid and refrigerate the sorbet mixture for at least 1-2 hours, or until thoroughly chilled.

Churn the Sorbet: Once chilled, transfer the sorbet mixture to an ice cream maker and churn according to the manufacturer's instructions, typically for about 20-25 minutes, or until it reaches a soft-serve consistency.

Freeze the Sorbet: Transfer the churned sorbet to a freezer-safe container and freeze for an additional 2-3 hours, or until firm.

Serve: Remove the sorbet from the freezer and let it soften slightly at room temperature for a few minutes before scooping. Serve the Coconut Mango Sorbet in bowls or cones, garnished with shredded coconut, fresh mint leaves, or lime zest, if desired.

Storage: You may keep any leftover sorbet in the freezer for up to one or two weeks by placing it in an airtight container. Before scooping and serving, let it soften for a few minutes at room temperature.

Nutritional Benefits:

Mangoes: Rich in vitamins A and C, potassium, fiber, and antioxidants, mangoes offer numerous health benefits, including improved immune function, digestion, and skin health.

Coconut Milk: Provides healthy fats, vitamins, and minerals, including medium-chain triglycerides (MCTs) that support brain health and metabolism. Coconut milk adds creaminess and a tropical flavor to the sorbet.

Lime Juice: Packed with vitamin C and antioxidants, lime juice adds tartness and brightness to the sorbet, enhancing the flavor of the mangoes and providing a refreshing contrast.

Natural Sweeteners: When used in moderation, natural sweeteners like sugar, agave nectar, or maple syrup offer sweetness without the added chemicals or refined sugar found in many commercial desserts.
Coconut Mango Sorbet is a delicious and guilt-free dessert option for vegetarians, offering a taste of the tropics in every scoop. Enjoy it as a refreshing treat on a hot day or as a light and fruity ending to any meal.

CHAPTER TEN

Beverages

Beverages on a vegetarian diet encompass a wide range of options that exclude meat and fish products but may include dairy, eggs, and other animal-derived ingredients. Here's a comprehensive explanation of various beverage options suitable for a vegetarian diet:

1. **Water:**
Water is the most essential beverage for hydration and overall health. It's calorie-free and essential for maintaining bodily functions, including digestion, nutrient absorption, temperature regulation, and waste elimination. Opt for filtered water to remove impurities and ensure quality. You can also infuse water with fruits, herbs, or cucumbers for added flavor and hydration.

2. **Plant-Based Milk:**

Plant-based milk alternatives are popular among vegetarians and vegans as dairy substitutes. Common options include almond milk, soy milk, oat milk, coconut milk, rice milk, and hemp milk.

Plant-based milk offers a variety of flavors and textures, suitable for drinking on its own, adding to cereal, coffee, tea, or using in cooking and baking.

Look for fortified plant-based milks that provide added nutrients like calcium, vitamin D, and vitamin B12 for a well-rounded diet.

3. **Fruit Juices:**

Fruit juices are made by extracting the liquid from fruits, providing vitamins, minerals, and antioxidants. Common options include orange juice, apple juice, grape juice, and pineapple juice.

While fruit juices can be a refreshing and tasty option, they can also be high in natural sugars and calories. Opt for freshly squeezed or 100% pure fruit juices without added sugars or preservatives for the healthiest choice.

4. Vegetable Juices:
Vegetable juices offer a nutrient-rich option for vegetarians, providing vitamins, minerals, and antioxidants from vegetables like carrots, beets, spinach, kale, and celery.
Green juices, in particular, are popular for their detoxifying properties and potential health benefits. You can make vegetable juices at home using a juicer or purchase them from health food stores or juice bars.

5. Smoothies:
Smoothies are blended beverages made with fruits, vegetables, plant-based milk, yogurt, and other ingredients. They offer a convenient and nutritious option for breakfast, snacks, or post-workout fuel.

Customize your smoothies with a variety of
ingredients like leafy greens, berries, bananas,
protein powder, nut butter, seeds, and spices
for added flavor and nutrition.
Avoid adding excessive sweeteners like sugar
or syrups to keep your smoothies healthy and
balanced.

6. **Tea:**

Tea is a popular beverage worldwide, offering a
variety of flavors, aromas, and health benefits.
Common types of tea include black tea, green
tea, white tea, oolong tea, and herbal tea.
Tea contains antioxidants, catechins, and other
compounds that may support heart health,
brain function, weight management, and
immunity.
Enjoy tea hot or cold, plain or with added
sweeteners, milk, lemon, or spices like ginger
or cinnamon for added flavor and warmth.

7. **Coffee:**
Coffee is a beloved beverage made from roasted coffee beans, providing caffeine and antioxidants. It's enjoyed by many vegetarians for its stimulating effects and rich flavor. Customize your coffee with milk or cream, sweeteners, flavored syrups, or spices like cinnamon or nutmeg to suit your taste preferences.
Be mindful of excessive caffeine consumption and its potential effects on sleep, anxiety, and digestion. Limit intake to moderate levels for optimal health.

8. **Nutritional Shakes:**
Nutritional shakes or meal replacement shakes are convenient options for vegetarians on the go. They typically contain protein, vitamins, minerals, and other nutrients, providing a balanced meal or snack in liquid form.

Look for plant-based nutritional shakes made from ingredients like pea protein, hemp protein, brown rice protein, and spirulina for a vegan-friendly option.

9. Alcoholic Beverages:

Alcoholic beverages like beer, wine, and spirits are generally considered vegetarian-friendly, although some products may use animal-derived ingredients or processing agents. Check labels or contact manufacturers for clarification.
Many breweries and wineries offer vegan-friendly options, and there are also dedicated vegan beer and wine brands available.

10. Specialty Beverages:

Specialty beverages encompass a wide range of options, including kombucha, coconut water, sports drinks, energy drinks, and health shots. These beverages offer unique flavors, functional benefits, and hydration options for vegetarians with diverse preferences.

Nutritional Considerations:
When selecting beverages on a vegetarian diet, it's essential to prioritize hydration and choose options that align with your health goals and dietary preferences.
Opt for whole food-based beverages whenever possible, such as water, herbal tea, or homemade smoothies, to maximize nutritional benefits and minimize added sugars, preservatives, and artificial ingredients.
Be mindful of portion sizes and added ingredients like sweeteners, syrups, and flavorings that can contribute to excess calories, sugar intake, and potential health risks.

Green Detox Smoothie

A Green Detox Smoothie is a nutritious and refreshing beverage made from a blend of leafy greens, fruits, and other wholesome ingredients. It's perfect for vegetarians looking to incorporate more plant-based foods into their diet while providing a burst of vitamins, minerals, fiber, and antioxidants. Here's a comprehensive explanation:

Ingredients:
Leafy Greens: Common leafy greens used in green detox smoothies include spinach, kale, Swiss chard, and collard greens. These greens are rich in vitamins (such as vitamin A, vitamin C, and vitamin K), minerals (such as iron, calcium, and magnesium), and antioxidants.

Fruits: Fruits add natural sweetness, flavor, and additional nutrients to the smoothie. Popular options include bananas, apples, pineapples, mangoes, kiwis, and berries. Fruits provide vitamins, minerals, fiber, and antioxidants essential for overall health.

Liquid Base: A liquid base like water, coconut water, almond milk, soy milk, or coconut milk helps thin out the smoothie and achieve the desired consistency. Choose unsweetened and unflavored options for a healthier choice.

Protein Source: Increasing the protein amount of the smoothie with Greek yogurt, tofu, or plant-based protein powder makes it more filling and nutritious. Protein helps with satiety, muscle growth, and repair.

Healthy Fats: Incorporating healthy fats like avocado, chia seeds, flaxseeds, or nut butter adds creaminess, richness, and satiety to the smoothie. Healthy fats provide essential fatty acids, vitamins, and antioxidants.

Optional Ingredients: You can customize your green detox smoothie with additional ingredients like fresh ginger, turmeric, mint leaves, lemon juice, cinnamon, or spirulina for added flavor, nutrition, and detoxifying properties.

Instructions:
Prepare Ingredients: Wash and chop the leafy greens and fruits as needed. Peel and core fruits like apples or pineapples if desired.

Mix well. components: Blend together the fruits, leafy greens, protein source, healthy fats, and any additional components in a blender. Blend until creamy and smooth, stopping occasionally to scrape down the blender's sides.

Modify Consistency: To thin out the smoothie to the appropriate consistency if it's too thick, add extra liquid base. Blend once more until completely integrated and smooth.

Taste and modify: Add extra fruits, sweeteners, or spices to the smoothie as needed to modify the sweetness or flavorings. Blend until completely combined once more.

Serve: Immediately serve the green detox smoothie by pouring it into glasses. For a touch of texture and presentation, garnish with almonds, seeds, nuts, or cinnamon.

Storage: You may keep any leftover smoothies in the fridge for up to one or two days by placing them in an airtight container. Before serving, give it a good shake or stir, as separation could happen.

Nutritional Benefits:

Leafy Greens: Rich in vitamins, minerals, fiber, and antioxidants, leafy greens support detoxification, digestion, immune function, and overall well-being.

Fruits: Provide natural sweetness, vitamins, minerals, fiber, and antioxidants, promoting hydration, digestion, and cellular health. Liquid Base: Hydrates the body, aids digestion, and supports nutrient absorption, providing essential fluids and electrolytes.

Protein Source: Supports muscle growth, repair, and satiety, helping maintain energy levels and muscle function.

Healthy Fats: Provide sustained energy, promote satiety, and support brain health, hormone production, and nutrient absorption.

A Green Detox Smoothie is a delicious and nutritious beverage option for vegetarians looking to boost their intake of fruits, vegetables, and plant-based ingredients. Enjoy it as a refreshing breakfast, snack, or post-workout refuel, knowing that it's packed with essential nutrients and detoxifying properties to support your health and well-being.

Watermelon Cucumber Cooler

A Watermelon Cucumber Cooler is a refreshing and hydrating beverage that's perfect for vegetarians seeking a light and flavorful option. Here's a comprehensive explanation:

Ingredients:
Watermelon: Fresh watermelon serves as the base of this cooler, providing natural sweetness, hydration, and a vibrant color. Watermelon is rich in vitamins (such as vitamin C and vitamin A), minerals (such as potassium), and antioxidants.

Cucumber: Cucumber adds a refreshing and crisp flavor to the cooler, complementing the sweetness of the watermelon. Cucumber is low in calories and rich in water, making it hydrating and refreshing.

Lime Juice: Lime juice adds brightness and acidity to the cooler, enhancing the flavors of the watermelon and cucumber. Lime juice also provides vitamin C and antioxidants.

Mint Leaves: Fresh mint leaves lend a cool and aromatic flavor to the cooler, adding a refreshing and herbaceous note. Mint leaves are known for their digestive properties and can help soothe the stomach.

Sweetener (Optional): To balance the flavors, you can add a sweetener like honey, agave nectar, or simple syrup, depending on how sweet the watermelon is. Depending on how sweet you desire, adjust the amount.

Ice: Ice cubes or crushed ice are added to the cooler to chill it and make it more refreshing. You can also freeze watermelon cubes or cucumber slices to use as ice cubes for added flavor.

Instructions:
Prepare Ingredients: Wash and dice the watermelon, discarding any seeds and rind. Peel and slice the cucumber into smaller pieces. Juice fresh limes to extract the lime juice. Pick fresh mint leaves from the stems.

Blend Ingredients: In a blender, combine the diced watermelon, sliced cucumber, lime juice, mint leaves, and optional sweetener. Blend until smooth and well combined.

Optional: To obtain a smoother texture and eliminate any pulp or seeds, pass the mixture through a fine-mesh sieve if you'd like. Depending on personal preference, this step can be skipped.

Chill: Transfer the strained mixture to a pitcher or serving container and refrigerate for at least 1-2 hours to chill and allow the flavors to meld together.

Serve: Once chilled, stir the cooler well and pour it into glasses filled with ice cubes. Garnish with fresh mint leaves or slices of cucumber or watermelon for a decorative touch.

Storage: You can keep any leftover Watermelon Cucumber Cooler in the refrigerator for up to a day or two by placing it in an airtight container. Before serving, give it a good stir because separation can happen.

Nutritional Benefits:
Watermelon: High in water content, watermelon provides hydration and electrolytes, making it a perfect summer fruit. It's also low in calories and packed with vitamins, minerals, and antioxidants, supporting overall health and hydration.

Cucumber: Similarly, cucumber is hydrating and low in calories, offering vitamins, minerals, and antioxidants. It aids digestion, promotes hydration, and adds a refreshing flavor to the cooler.

Lime Juice: Rich in vitamin C and antioxidants, lime juice supports immune function, collagen production, and skin health. It adds acidity and brightness to the cooler, enhancing the flavors of the other ingredients.

Mint Leaves: Mint leaves provide a refreshing and cooling sensation, aiding digestion and freshening breath. They add a pleasant herbal note to the cooler, making it more flavorful and aromatic.

Golden Tumeric Latte

A Golden Turmeric Latte, also known as a Golden Milk Latte, is a warm and comforting beverage with a vibrant golden hue, made from turmeric and other wholesome ingredients. It's a popular drink among vegetarians and those seeking a dairy-free alternative to traditional lattes. Here's a comprehensive explanation:

Ingredients:

Turmeric: Turmeric is the star ingredient of the latte, providing its distinctive golden color and earthy flavor. Turmeric contains curcumin, a compound with anti-inflammatory and antioxidant properties, offering potential health benefits.

Milk: Plant-based milk like almond milk, coconut milk, soy milk, oat milk, or cashew milk serves as the base of the latte. Choose unsweetened and unflavored options for a healthier choice. Plant-based milk provides calcium, vitamins, and minerals while being dairy-free.

Sweetener: To counterbalance the bitterness of the turmeric, a natural sweetener like honey, maple syrup, agave nectar, or coconut sugar adds sweetness to the latte. Depending on how sweet you desire, adjust the amount.

Spices: Additional spices like cinnamon, ginger, black pepper, and cardamom are often added to the latte for flavor complexity and added health benefits. These spices offer warmth, depth, and digestive support.

Optional Ingredients: You can customize your Golden Turmeric Latte with additional ingredients like vanilla extract, coconut oil, or collagen powder for added flavor, creaminess, or nutritional benefits.

Guidelines:
Get ready Ingredients: Scoop out the sweetener, spices, and turmeric. Peel and coarsely grate fresh ginger if using it.

Warm Milk: Heat the plant-based milk in a small saucepan over medium-low heat until it's warm but not boiling. Stir from time to time to avoid burning.

Mix well. Ingredients: To make a paste, put the turmeric, sugar, spices, and a tiny bit of heated milk in a blender or mixing bowl. This guarantees that the spices are dispersed uniformly.

Mix with Milk: Whisk or blend continually until the spice paste is smooth and well integrated. Slowly add the remaining heated milk to the paste.

Warm and Simmer: Transfer the blend back into the saucepan and gently warm it on low heat, stirring continuously, until the latte gets hot and frothy. Take care not to allow it to boil.

Taste and Adjust: If necessary, adjust the latte's sweetness or spice level. To suit your taste, increase the amount of spices or sweetener.

To serve, immediately transfer the Golden Turmeric Latte into mugs. For extra taste and visual appeal, garnish with a cinnamon stick or a dusting of ground cinnamon.

Storage: You can keep any leftover lattes in the fridge for two to three days by placing them in an airtight container. Before serving, gently reheat in the microwave or on the stove.

Nutritional Benefits:
Turmeric: Contains curcumin, a powerful anti-inflammatory and antioxidant compound that may offer numerous health benefits, including reduced inflammation, improved digestion, and enhanced immune function.

Plant-Based Milk: Provides calcium, vitamins, and minerals while being dairy-free and lactose-free. Plant-based milk supports bone health, muscle growth, and overall well-being.

Spices: Cinnamon, ginger, black pepper, and cardamom offer additional antioxidant properties, digestive support, and warming effects, enhancing the flavor and health benefits of the latte.

Natural Sweeteners: When used in moderation, natural sweeteners like honey, maple syrup, or agave nectar offer sweetness without the added chemicals or refined sugar found in many commercial drinks.

A Golden Turmeric Latte is a delicious and nutritious beverage option for vegetarians seeking a warming and healing drink. Enjoy it as a soothing treat on a chilly day or as a comforting bedtime drink, knowing that it's packed with wholesome ingredients and potential health benefits.

CONCLUSION

In conclusion, the Vegetarian Diet Cookbook 2024 offers a comprehensive collection of delicious and nutritious recipes tailored to the needs and preferences of individuals following a vegetarian diet. From vibrant salads to hearty soups, flavorful mains, and indulgent desserts, this cookbook showcases the versatility and abundance of plant-based ingredients.

Throughout the cookbook, we have explored a wide range of vegetarian-friendly dishes, each highlighting the benefits of incorporating more fruits, vegetables, whole grains, legumes, nuts, and seeds into our daily meals. These recipes not only nourish the body but also tantalize the taste buds, proving that vegetarian cuisine can be satisfying, flavorful, and enjoyable for everyone.

Whether you're a seasoned vegetarian looking for new culinary inspirations or someone curious about adopting a more plant-based lifestyle, this cookbook provides a wealth of options to suit every palate and occasion. From quick and easy weeknight dinners to impressive dishes for special gatherings, there's something for every meal and mood.

We've delved into the health benefits of key ingredients used in vegetarian cooking, highlighting their nutritional value and potential contributions to overall well-being. From leafy greens packed with vitamins and antioxidants to plant-based proteins supporting muscle health and fiber-rich grains promoting digestive health, each ingredient plays a vital role in supporting a balanced and wholesome diet.

Moreover, the cookbook emphasizes the importance of mindful eating, sustainability, and ethical considerations associated with vegetarianism. By choosing plant-based foods, we not only nourish our bodies but also reduce our environmental footprint and support animal welfare, contributing to a healthier planet for future generations.

In essence, the Vegetarian Diet Cookbook 2024 serves as a comprehensive guide and culinary companion for anyone interested in exploring the vibrant and diverse world of vegetarian cuisine. With its enticing recipes, nutritional insights, and practical tips, this cookbook empowers individuals to embrace a plant-based lifestyle and discover the joys of vegetarian cooking. Cheers to delicious, nutritious, and compassionate eating!

Thank you for embarking on this culinary journey with the Vegetarian Diet Cookbook 2024. Your decision to explore the vibrant world of plant-based cuisine not only nourishes your body but also supports a healthier planet and a more compassionate way of living.

By choosing vegetarian meals, you are making a positive impact on your health, the environment, and animal welfare. With every delicious recipe you try, you are taking a step towards a more sustainable and ethical way of eating.

We hope this cookbook has inspired you to discover new flavors, experiment with wholesome ingredients, and embrace the joys of vegetarian cooking. Together, let's continue to celebrate the abundance of plant-based foods and create a brighter, greener future for ourselves and generations to come.

Thank you for being part of the Vegetarian Diet Cookbook 2024 journey. Happy cooking, happy eating, and happy living!